nics.com

NURSING CLINICS
OF NORTH AMERICA

Pharmacology

GUEST EDITOR
Suzanne S. Prevost, PhD, RN, CNAA

March 2005 • Volume 40 • Number 1

SAUNDERS

An Imprint of Elsevier, Inc.
PHILADELPHIA   LONDON   TORONTO   MONTREAL   SYDNEY   TOKYO

W.B. SAUNDERS COMPANY

A Division of Elsevier Inc.

The Curtis Center • Independence Square West • Philadelphia, Pennsylvania 19106

http://www.theclinics.com

THE NURSING CLINICS OF NORTH AMERICA
March 2005
Editor: Maria Lorusso

Volume 40, Number 1
ISSN 0029-6465
ISBN 1-4160-2736-X

The ideas and opinions expressed in *The Nursing Clinics of North America* do not necessarily reflect those of the Publisher. The Publisher does not assume any responsibility for any injury and/ or damage to persons or property arising out of or related to any use of the material contained in this periodical. The reader is advised to check the appropriate medical literature and the product information currently provided by the manufacturer of each drug to be administered to verify the dosage, the method and duration of administration, or contraindications. It is the responsibility of the treating physician or other health care professional, relying on independent experience and knowledge of the patient, to determine drug dosages and the best treatment for the patient. Mention of any product in this issue should not be construed as endorsement by the contributors, editors, or the Publisher of the product or manufacturers' claims.

The Nursing Clinics of North America (ISSN 0029-6465) is published quarterly by Elsevier Inc., Corporate and Editorial Offices: Elsevier Inc., 170 S Independence Mall W 300 E, Philadelphia, PA 19106-3399. Accounting and Circulation Offices: 6277 Sea Harbor Drive, Orlando, FL 32887-4800. Periodicals postage paid at Orlando, FL 32862, and additional mailing offices. Subscription price per year is, $100.00 (US individuals), $191.00 (US institutions), $165.00 (international individuals), $225.00 (international institutions), $138.00 (Canadian individuals), $225.00 (Canadian institutions), $55.00 (US students), and $83.00 (international students). To receive student/resident rate, orders must be accompanied by name of affiliated institution, date of term, and the signature of program/residency coordinator on institution letterhead. Orders will be billed at individual rate until proof of status is received. Foreign air speed delivery is included in all *Clinics* subscription prices. All prices are subject to change without notice. POSTMASTER: Send address changes to W.B. Saunders Company, Periodicals Fulfillment, Orlando, FL 32887-4800. **Customer Service: 1-800-654-2452 (US). From outside of the US, call 1-407-345-4000.**

Nursing Clinics of North America is covered in *EMBASE/Excerpta Medica, Index Medicus, Social Sciences Citation Index, Current Contents, ASCA, Cumulative Index to Nursing, RNdex Top 100,* and *Allied Health Literature and International Nursing Index (INI).*

Printed in the United States of America.

GUEST EDITOR

SUZANNE S. PREVOST, PhD, RN, CNAA, Professor and National HealthCare Chair of Excellence, School of Nursing, Middle Tennessee State University, Murfreesboro, Tennessee

CONTRIBUTORS

ROXANNE K. BOWMAN, BSN, RN, Graduate Research Assistant, Pediatric Nurse Practitioner Program, College of Nursing, University of Kentucky, Lexington, Kentucky

PATRICIA V. BURKHART, PhD, RN, Assistant Professor, College of Nursing, University of Kentucky, Lexington, Kentucky

LINDA W. COVINGTON, PhD, RN, Professor, School of Nursing, Middle Tennessee State University, Murfreesboro, Tennessee

ANITA B. CROCKETT, PhD, RN, Associate Professor, School of Nursing, Middle Tennessee State University, Murfreesboro, Tennessee

ROBIN DONOHOE DENNISON, RN, MSN, CCNS, Doctoral Student, University of Kentucky College of Nursing, Lexington, Kentucky; and Critical Care Nursing Consultant, Winchester, Kentucky

KEN W. EDMISSON, ND, EdD, RNC, FNP, Associate Professor, School of Nursing, Middle Tennessee State University, Murfreesboro, Tennessee

KATHY HAIG, RN, Director, Quality Resource Management; Patient Safety Officer; and Risk Manager, OSF St. Joseph Medical Center, Bloomington, Illinois

ROBERTA KAPLOW, RN, PhD, CCNS, CCRN, Clinical Professor, Nell Hodgson Woodruff School of Nursing, Emory University, Atlanta, Georgia

KATHY J. MORRIS, RN, MSN, ARNP, FNP-BC, Family Practice Nurse Practitioner, Council Bluffs Community Health Center, Council Bluffs, Iowa

LYNN C. PARSONS, DSN, RN, CNA, Professor and Director, School of Nursing, Middle Tennessee State University, Murfreesboro, Tennessee

MARY KAY RAYENS, PhD, Associate Professor, Colleges of Nursing and Medicine, University of Kentucky, Lexington, Kentucky

TOM RONE, RN, CCRN, Patient Care Director, Intensive Care Unit, Middle Tennessee Medical Center, Murfreesboro, Tennessee

JENNY L. SAULS, DSN, RN, C, Associate Professor of Nursing, School of Nursing, Middle Tennessee State University, Murfreesboro, Tennessee

DEBORAH S. SMITH, RN, MS, MBA, CNAA, Assistant Administrator, Patient Services; Chief Nurse Executive, OSF St. Joseph Medical Center, Bloomington, Illinois

MARIA A. SMITH, DSN, RN, CCRN, Professor, School of Nursing, Middle Tennessee State University, Murfreesboro, Tennessee

KAREN S. WARD, PhD, RN, COI, Professor and Associate Director, Online Programs, School of Nursing, Middle Tennessee State University, Murfreesboro, Tennessee

CONTRIBUTORS

CONTENTS

Medical and nursing students have traditionally been taught Hippocrates' dictum first do no harm. Unfortunately, unintentional patient harm at the hands of health care professionals has been the focus of recent studies, national investigations, and public attention. In the mid-1990s, several medical incidents that resulted in serious adverse consequences to patients were highly publicized, stimulating the interest and concern of the public and health care professionals regarding the safety of the health care system. The estimated financial cost of medical errors in the United States is approximately $37.6 billion each year, with $17 billion of these costs associated with preventable errors. One third of all medical errors involve medication errors, making these the most common cause of preventable medical errors.

This article discusses the experiences of a community hospital on the path to improved patient safety. It focuses specifically on efforts to reduce adverse drug events through initiatives in developing a culture of safety. Tactics focus on creating the safety culture, medication reconciliation, failure mode effects analysis, controlled use of high-risk medications, and the use of standardized order sets.

prescribing antibiotics, use of hygiene measures and nonpharmacologic treatments, and continued surveillance.

Innovations in Antineoplastic Therapy

Roberta Kaplow

Innovations in the treatment of cancer are developed on a regular basis. The US Food and Drug Administration (FDA) frequently makes announcements about agents approved for either clinical trials or clinician use as part of the arsenal against cancer. Ongoing research in the basic sciences has led to an enhanced understanding of cancer. This knowledge has resulted in new key scientific advances to combat disease. This article reviews the antineoplastic therapies that have received FDA approval within the past 3 years.

New Developments in Antidepressant Therapy

Karen S. Ward

Depression is an overwhelmingly common problem in the United States. It is not only life threatening, but also costly, both personally and financially. Following a brief overview of depression, this article presents a variety of treatment modalities. Advantages and disadvantages of each intervention are explored along with suggestions for evaluating current and future advances in treatment options.

Multidimensional Pharmacologic Strategies for Diabetes

Ken W. Edmisson

Managing diabetes and its complications has become one of this country's largest health concerns. Diabetes care is complex and requires a multi-faceted approach including lifestyle management, diet and exercise, management of comorbid illnesses, and meticulous pharmacologic interventions. New guidelines for diabetes management have been established to provide for better health in patients who have diabetes.

Osteoporosis: Incidence, Prevention, and Treatment of the Silent Killer

Lynn C. Parsons

Osteoporosis is a significant health care concern for millions of Americans. This disease is characterized by low bone mass and deterioration of bone tissue, which can lead to fractures. Ten million Americans suffer from osteoporosis and another 34 million are estimated to have osteopenia (ie, low bone mass) which places them at greater risk for osteoporosis. Osteoporosis is often thought of as a disease that affects only older women, but osteoporosis can occur at any age and in either gender. This article focuses on the incidence, prevention, and treatment of this "silent killer," and current pharmacologic advances are reviewed, including vitamin and mineral therapies.

Heart failure is a serious condition in which the heart does not pump well enough to meet the oxygenation needs of the body. Millions of people suffer from this debilitating disease, and despite advances in treatment, 50% of those diagnosed die within five years. Current research indicates that beta blockers, specifically bisoprolol, metoprolol, and carvedilol, actually reduce morbidity and mortality of heart failure. Current guidelines published by the Heart Failure Society of America recommend the use of beta blocking drugs for the treatment of patients suffering with mild to severe symptoms of heart failure. These drugs should be used as a cornerstone of therapy in combination with diuretics and angiotensin-converting enzyme inhibitors to increase the quality of life for these patients.

The diagnosis and treatment of patients who have HIV and AIDS is challenging for most nurses. New pharmaceutic therapies, which are vital components of care for these individuals, are constantly evolving. Issues from weight loss and gain, heart disease, insulin resistance, and even increased bone metabolism must be considered when determining appropriate pharmaceutic regimens. New complications often arise with new treatments; living longer may not always mean living better. Use of appropriate drug therapy and management of individual drug implications can help patients who have HIV and AIDS live longer and enjoy a better quality of life.

Children's metered-dose inhaler (MDI) technique for asthma medications was evaluated pre- and postteaching. A majority (92%) of the children (N = 36) used their MDIs incorrectly during the pretest. The most common mistakes were: (1) not holding breath after actuation, (2) not waiting between inhalations, (3) inadequately shaking the medication, (4) not inhaling the medication fully, and (5) not using a spacer. The children made significant improvement in their MDI technique after receiving instruction ($P < 0.001$). The results of this study underscore the importance of teaching and reinforcing accurate medication administration technique at each health encounter.

FORTHCOMING ISSUES

RECENT ISSUES

THE CLINICS ARE NOW AVAILABLE ONLINE!

Access your subscription at:
http://www.theclinics.com

NURSING
CLINICS
OF NORTH AMERICA

Nurs Clin N Am 40 (2005) xi–xii

Preface

Pharmacology

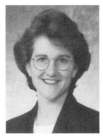

Suzanne S. Prevost, PhD, RN, CNAA
Guest Editor

Although medication management is a fundamental nursing responsibility, staying abreast of new pharmacologic developments can seem overwhelming. Over 8000 pharmaceutical products are on the market today [1]. Every month new drugs are released and the knowledge related to existing drugs evolves with the identification of new indications, new adverse effects, and new opportunities to help or harm consumers. Nurses in every role and specialty, from direct caregivers in hospitals to nurse practitioners in primary care clinics, are continuously challenged to maintain and expand their knowledge of medications.

Many nursing students struggle just to grasp a basic understanding of drug classifications and the implications for the most frequently administered therapies. The real understanding evolves as nurses gain clinical experience and repeated exposure to the common drugs in their areas of specialization. Yet even the most experienced nurse must commit to lifelong learning to stay ahead of today's knowledgeable health care consumers.

Important pharmaceutical research often hits the newspapers before it is covered in nursing journals and texts. Patients and families come to the health care setting armed with the latest drug news, direct-to-consumer drug advertisements, and Internet searches of their diagnoses and prescriptions. Those patients and families often judge nursing competence on the basis of the nurses' knowledge, skill, and speed in administering medications. These trends compound the need for continuing nursing education related to pharmaceuticals.

0029-6465/05/$ - see front matter © 2005 Elsevier Inc. All rights reserved.
doi:10.1016/j.cnur.2004.11.001 **nursing.theclinics.com**

In this issue of the *Nursing Clinics of North America*, we offer a broad sample of new developments in pharmacology. Because medication safety and error prevention are high priorities for nurses, administrators, payers, and patients, we begin with Dennison's comprehensive review of strategies for promoting medication safety. Smith then shares a case study describing her institution's success in reducing adverse drug events. Crockett provides a thought-provoking analysis of prescribing patterns. Morris offers practical advice to help senior citizens address their top public policy concern: acquiring affordable medications. Topical articles provide updates on recent developments in several specific drug classifications from antibiotics and antineoplastics to antidepressants. Drugs for specific illnesses, including diabetes, osteoporosis, heart failure and AIDS, are also covered. Finally, Burkhart, Rayens, and Bowman share their research findings and clinical implications related to children's use of metered-dose inhalers for asthma medications.

It would be impossible to cover the entire scope of new pharmacologic developments in a single issue. We offer this collection of articles in the hope that nurses from a broad spectrum of roles and specialties will find new and practical information to expand their knowledge and enhance their care of patients and their families.

Suzanne S. Prevost, PhD, RN, CNAA
Professor and National HealthCare Chair of Excellence
School of Nursing
Middle Tennessee State University
Murfreesboro, TN 37132, USA

E-mail address: sprevost@mtsu.edu

Reference

[1] Low DK, Belcher JV. Reporting medication errors through computerized medication administration. CIN. Comput Inform Nurs 2002;20:178–83.

ELSEVIER
SAUNDERS

NURSING
CLINICS
OF NORTH AMERICA

Nurs Clin N Am 40 (2005) 1–23

Creating an Organizational Culture for Medication Safety

Robin Donohoe Dennison, RN, MSN, CCNS[a,b]

[a]*University of Kentucky College of Nursing, Lexington, KY, USA*
[b]*Critical Care Nursing Consultant, 108 Hidden Grove Lane, Winchester, KY 40391, USA*

Description of the problem

Medical and nursing students have traditionally been taught Hippocrates' dictum *first do no harm*. Unfortunately, unintentional patient harm at the hands of health care professionals has been the focus of recent studies, national investigations, and public attention [1]. In the mid-1990s, several medical incidents that resulted in serious adverse consequences to patients were highly publicized, stimulating the interest and concern of the public and health care professionals regarding the safety of the health care system [2]. In 2000, the Institute of Medicine (IOM) focused national attention on the incidence, consequences, and cost of medical errors, including those involving medication, with the publication of *To Err is Human: Building a Safer Health System* [1].

The IOM defines error as "the failure of a planned action to be completed as intended or the use of a wrong plan to achieve an aim" and estimates that between 44,000 and 98,000 Americans die each year as a result of medical errors [1]. The estimated financial cost of medical errors in the United States is approximately $37.6 billion each year, with $17 billion of these costs associated with preventable errors [1]. One third of all medical errors involve medication errors, making these the most common cause of preventable medical errors [3].

A medication error is defined as "any preventable event that may cause or lead to inappropriate medication use or patient harm while the medication is in the control of the health care professional, patient, or consumer" [4]. The error "may be related to professional practice, health care products, procedures, and systems, including prescribing; order communication;

E-mail address: robin@robindennison.com

product labeling, packaging, and nomenclature; compounding; dispensing; distribution; administration; education; monitoring; and use" [4].

Adverse drug event (ADE) is another term that is frequently used, especially in the medicine and pharmacy literature, to refer to incidents when the patient is harmed by a drug [5]. This term is more comprehensive than "medication errors" because it includes harm as a result of an error in addition to adverse reactions such as rash, anaphylaxis, nephrotoxicity, hepatotoxicity, or blood dyscrasias. About one third of ADEs are associated with medication errors and are therefore considered preventable [6]. Potential ADE refers to an error that was caught before it reached the patient, but could have harmed the patient if the drug had actually been administered. These are also frequently referred to as *near misses*.

Bates et al [7] found that medication errors occur at a rate of 5 per 100 medication doses. Fortunately, not all errors cause patient harm. Only 7% of medication errors have significant potential for patient harm and only 1% actually result in patient harm [5]. Therefore, for every medication error that harms a patient, there are 100 that do not [8]. Unfortunately, many of the errors that do not cause harm are not detected, and of those that are detected, many are not reported. According to the IOM report, medication errors affect 3% to 5% of patients [1,9] and cause more than 7000 deaths annually [1].

Medication errors are costly from human, economic, and societal perspectives. From the human perspective, patients may suffer discomfort, complications, prolonged hospitalization, disability, or death, whereas the health care professional responsible for the error frequently suffers severe emotional distress. Nurses frequently equate errors with harm to the patient and failure of their moral and ethical responsibility to "do no harm" [10].

Serembus et al [11] found that health care professionals involved in a fatal medication error not only remembered the details of the error but also experienced consequent feelings of guilt and sadness. The researchers identified several standard responses to the experience of making a fatal medication error, including: (1) feeling of responsibility for the patient's death, (2) acknowledgment of failure, (3) fear of punishment, (4) desire to correct the wrong, (5) denial of personal accountability, (6) guilt and depression about the death, (7) perception of public humiliation, (8) need for support, (9) coping, (10) fatalism, and (11) concern about the likelihood of future errors.

The economic impact of medication errors affects individuals, health care organizations, third-party payers, and society. In a study by Bates and colleagues [12], the economic impact of medication errors was found to be $4685 per error, or an annual cost of $2.8 million for a 700-bed teaching hospital. This was a conservative estimate because it did not include the cost of injuries to the patient, admissions caused by drug errors, malpractice litigation, or additional labor caused by the patient's increased needs. The occurrence of an adverse drug event was associated with an average increased length of stay of 1.91 days in a study conducted by Classen and colleagues [13], and 2.2 days in the study by Bates et al [12]. The cost of drug-related morbidity and mortality is estimated to be more than $136 billion a year in the United States [14]. This financial burden affects the cost of health care, health insurance, and the profitability and even potential survival of many health care organizations, especially small and independent community hospitals.

In 1995, the American Nurses Association developed the Nursing Report Card for Acute Care Setting, which listed medication errors as one of five outcomes closely linked to quality of care and in need of improvement [15]. The second most common reason for malpractice litigation against nurses is medication errors, and the administration of medications is one of the highest risk areas of nursing practice [16] because errors made by nurses are much more likely to actually reach the patient. Errors made in the ordering phase are intercepted 48% to 70% of the time [6,17], whereas errors made during the administration phase have essentially no chance of being intercepted [6]. Errors made by the physician are likely to be intercepted either by the pharmacist or the nurse, and errors made by the pharmacist are often intercepted by the nurse, but it is unlikely that errors made by the nurse will be intercepted. Therefore, these errors have the most potential to harm the patient. The series of human checks is frequently referred to as a "human safety net" [18], but because this system is inadequate at the nursing level where medications are commonly dispensed, it is desirable for nurses to have a safety net established at the point of drug administration, most effectively in the form of technology.

Leape [17] found that 39% of medication errors occurred during physician ordering, 38% during a nurse's administration of a drug, 12% during transcription, and 11% during pharmacy dispensing (Fig. 1). Olsen [19] notes that nearly half of all medication errors occur during the prescribing process, causing errors downstream in dispensing or administration of the drug. Types of medication errors have been studied extensively and the results show significant variation (Fig. 2).

Patients who are sicker, subjected to multiple interventions, and remain in the hospital longer are more likely to suffer serious injury as a result of medical error [20]. Wilson and colleagues [21] found a greater risk of death and greater number of preventable adverse events associated with patients with complex cases, illnesses requiring urgent care, and the use of interventions thought to be potentially lifesaving. Weingart and colleagues [20] note that certain interventions, such as cardiothoracic surgery, vascular surgery, and neurosurgery increase the risk for error. But even though there are higher-risk patients, all patients are vulnerable to error.

Even with 99% accuracy rates, mortality and morbidity of patients is above acceptable levels. What is the acceptable level? Is it Six Sigma (ie, 99.99976% accuracy rate) or is it zero (ie, 100% accuracy rate)? Although some people apply the principles of Six Sigma to health care [22,23], Cooper [24] argues that whereas zero defects is an appropriate challenge and goal, we must recognize that humans will always err.

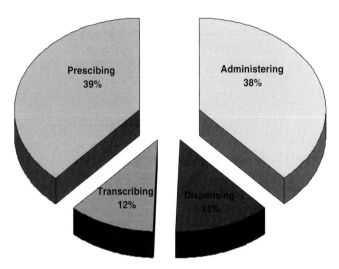

Fig. 1. Medication errors: stage of occurrence. *Data from* Leape LL. System analysis of adverse drug events. JAMA 1995;274(1):25–43.

The inevitability of human error

Traditional approaches to the reduction of medication errors have primarily focused on the individual, based on the belief that errors occur as a result of carelessness, forgetfulness, and negligence [18]. Disciplinary action for the individual who committed the error has been the typical response to a medication error, along with training, retraining, and remediation initiatives to inculcate the "five rights" (ie, right patient, right drug, right dose, right time, and right route) [17]. This punitive approach has reduced the reporting of medication errors, thereby increasing the potential risk to

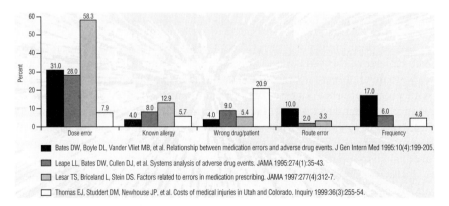

Fig. 2. Commonly studied medication errors as cause of ADEs: percentage of ADEs for each cause. *Data from* US Department of Health and Human Services. Reducing and preventing ADEs to decrease hospital costs. Available at: www.ahrq.gov/qual/aderia/aderia.htm. Accessed November 7, 2003.

the patient and inhibiting opportunities to correct the many system factors that contributed to the error. Because human error is unavoidable, this person-focused approach impedes the problem-solving process and prevents improvement in patient safety [25].

A major consequence of punishment for errors has been the reluctance to report medication errors. National surveys reveal that actual error rates are 38% higher than reported error rates [26]. The major reason that nurses cite for underreporting errors is fear of punitive action [27,28]. Gladstone [29] found that a large percentage of nurses believed that fear of disciplinary action prevented all errors from being reported, especially minor errors.

Weingart and colleagues [20] report that despite rare examples of malevolent providers, there is little evidence that medical errors are due to "bad apples." Consistent with that perception, Murphy [30] found that the age, educational level, and assignment of registered nurses who were disciplined for medication errors were no different from those of the registered nurse population as a whole. Anderson and Webster [25] claim that it is very unlikely for a nurse to retire without ever making a medication error, although the fortunate nurses will have not harmed a patient.

The IOM report emphasized that most medical errors are systems-related and not attributable to individual negligence or misconduct. The report stressed that the cause of medical errors is not bad people, but that "good people are working in bad systems" [1]. Nevertheless, in a recent survey of nurses, 79% believed it was true that "most medication errors occur when a nurse carelessly neglects to follow the five rights of medication administration."[31] Medication errors in nursing have traditionally been dealt with by nonsystematic, punitive, and ineffective means, with little knowledge of or attention to the factors that caused errors to occur. The current focus, therefore, is on a systems approach to include understanding and addressing the contributing factors underlying an error [25]. Processes that worked decades ago no longer ensure safe care in today's complex and highly technical health care system. The key to reducing medical errors is to focus on improving the health care delivery systems rather than to assign blame [1].

Crane [32] proposed three major steps to change the way medication errors and the medication use cycle are considered. First of all, the error reporting system should not be used for punishment. There also needs to be recognition that the current approaches to preventing medication errors are inadequate. Finally, a greater understanding of human performance in the medication use process needs to be developed and strategies identified that enhance rather than restrict human performance.

Rasmussen and Jensen [33] describe a model of performance that it based on the concept of cognition, which national medical errors expert Lucian Leape believes is particularly well-suited for analysis of errors [34]. In this model, human performance is classified into three levels: skill-based, rule-based, and knowledge-based. Skill-based performance is largely unconscious and governed by stored patterns of preprogrammed instructions.

Rule-based performance is governed by remembered rules to familiar problems (eg, if X, then Y). Knowledge-based performance requires conscious analytical thought and the use of stored knowledge to solve novel situations. Skill-based errors are caused by glitches in automatic activity and are referred to as *slips*. Rule-based and knowledge-based errors are caused by errors in conscious thought and are referred to as *mistakes*. [33]. Kelly [35], summarizing more than 1500 published case reports of ADE from 1976 through 1997, found that medication errors were categorized as a mistake 66% of the time and as a slip 34% of the time.

Reason [36] notes that "fallibility is part of the human condition" and states that although we can't change our fallibility, we can change the conditions of the work environment so that the potential for errors is reduced and the damaging effects of errors that do occur are contained. Reason's Organizational Accident Model (Fig. 3) examines the events up to an accident (or error), considers the actions of involved individuals, and then analyzes the working conditions and the organizational context in which the accident occurred.

Reason writes that human decisions or actions may contribute to adverse events through latent or active failures [37]. Latent failures arise from decisions made by people not directly involved in the immediate point of care, such as the management team. These decisions may cause difficulties for the clinical staff in the form of inadequate communication systems, heavy workloads, poor skill-mix, insufficient training or supervision, and inadequate or defective equipment. Active failures are unsafe acts committed by people involved at the immediate point of care (commonly referred to as the *sharp end*). These active failures include action slips (eg, picking up the wrong vial), cognitive failures (eg, not knowing, not remembering, or misinterpreting), and deviations from safe practices, procedures, and standards and can have immediate consequences [38].

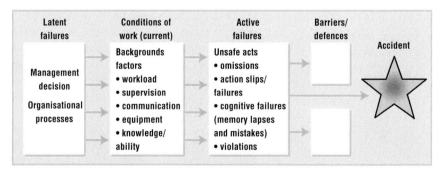

Fig. 3. Organizational accident model. *From* Reason J. Understanding adverse events: human factors. In: Vincent C, editor. Clinical risk management. London: BMJ Pubishing Group; 1995:31–54; with permission.

Reason [39] has also proposed the "Swiss Cheese Model of System Accidents" (Fig. 4). Defenses, barriers, and safeguards are built into our health care systems to protect the patient from human error. These safeguards may be human, technical, or procedural. Consider that even though these defenses are usually effective, each one has inherent weakness (ie, latent and active failures). Fortunately, one weakness does not allow an error to occur. However, when there is concurrent failure of all of the defenses, error and potential patient harm can occur. Reason advocates creating systems that are better able to tolerate the occurrence of single or even multiple errors and contain the effects to limit the consequences to the patient. With the recognition of the inevitability of human error comes the need for adequate safety net systems. A well-designed safety net does not allow an error to reach the patient unless several errors occur.

Pronovost and colleagues [40] advocate a three-pronged approach to patient safety: (1) prevent the error from occurring, (2) raise awareness of an error if it does occur (eg, immediate and accurate reporting of errors and near misses), (3) be better able to diminish harm to the patient should an error occur. Health care providers, being human, will not be able to perform without errors even in a well-designed medication delivery system. Therefore, establishing processes to learn from errors and minimize injury to the patient is vital.

Organizational culture of safety

Organizational culture represents the "shared beliefs, values, norms, expectations, and assumptions that are manifested in behavior and that bind

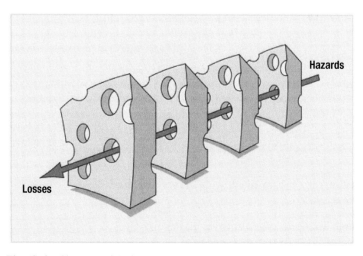

Fig. 4. The "Swiss Cheese Model of System Accidents." *From* Reason J. Human error: models and management. BMJ 2000;320:768–70; with permission.

people to the organization" [41]. It is the way the members in an organization behave and the values that are important to them, and may be described as "the way we do things here" or a way of life [42,43]. The IOM report identifies a need to create cultures of safety within all health care organizations [1]. Cooper [44] writes that a culture of safety is the result of effective interplay of environment structure and processes, attitude and perception of workers, and behavior related to safety.

The health care organization must be a learning environment to build and maintain a culture of safety. Error reporting should be confidential and exist without fear of blame [45]. Reporting should include near misses. Valuable quantitative analysis of near misses is possible because these potential ADEs occur much more frequently than actual errors [46]. Learning from errors and near misses prevents history from repeating itself in potentially devastating ways.

Four characteristics that can inhibit the change to a culture of safety were identified during the 2001 Quality Interagency Coordination Task Force. These include: (1) medicine's tendency to view errors as failure and warrant blame, (2) nurse training which frequently emphasizes rules rather than knowledge, (3) corrective actions focused on the person rather than the system, and (4) a "no blood, no foul" mentality which assumes no harm if the patient has not been injured [47].

A barrier to developing a culture of safety is an environment with unrealistic expectations of clinical perfection [45]. Leape [34] writes that efforts at error prevention have characteristically followed what might be called the perfectibility model, where the underlying belief is that "if physicians and nurses could be properly trained and motivated then they would make no mistakes." This goal of clinical perfection causes shame and guilt when an error occurs and discourages reporting [28,48–51]. In a recent survey of nurses, 58% responded that the statement, "error reporting is a valuable tool to measure a nurse's medication competency" was accurate [31]. Litigation practices and regulatory boards reinforce this perfectibility model [45]. Therefore, an anonymous system for reporting errors and near misses would significantly improve reporting practices. Disciplinary actions, job termination, loss of licensure, and malpractice litigation are powerful disincentives to reporting medication errors. An important organizational goal should be to create a culture that accepts the fallibility of humans and solicits the assistance of team members in the development of safeguards for error prevention.

Interventions to prevent medication errors and limit the consequences of medication errors

Though many interventions have been proposed to prevent medication errors or to limit the consequences of medication errors should they occur, most of these interventions have not been empirically tested. Nursing research has been focused primarily on the frequency of medication errors, the perceived causes of medication errors, the causes and significance of reporting deficiencies, the best teaching methods for information regarding drug safety and medication calculations, and the impact of the commission of a medication error on the nurse. Proposed interventions to create an organizational culture for medication safety are summarized by the PATIENT SAFE taxonomy (Table 1). This taxonomy provides a brief description of each intervention and its level of evidence. Note that more research is needed to evaluate many of the proposed interventions.

Patient involvement

In a survey conducted by the American Society of Health-System Pharmacists, 61% of Americans were "very concerned" about being given the wrong drug and 58% were "very concerned" about being given drugs that would interact in a negative way [52]. Aspden and colleagues [53] identify involvement of patients and their families as a key aspect of a patient safety program and write that patients represent the last point of error detection and prevention. Furthermore, medication administration time provides a "teachable moment," allowing the nurse to teach the patient the name of the drug, why it has been prescribed, what it does, and any adverse effects to expect or report [54].

Some specific ways that patients can contribute to safe medication therapy include keeping health care professionals informed and becoming educated about their own specific health problems and therapies. The National Patient Safety Foundation, the Agency for Health care Research and Quality, and the Institute for Safe Medication Practice have all developed materials to instruct patients about what they can do to improve the safety of health care [53].

Table 1
"PATIENT SAFE" taxonomy for drug safety

	Intervention	Level of evidence
P	Patient involvement	D
A	Adherence to established policies and procedures	C
T	Technology use	B
I	Information accessibility	C
E	Education regarding drug safety	D
N	Nonpunitive approach to reporting of errors and near misses	D
T	Teamwork, communication, and collaboration	B
S	Staffing	B
A	Administrative support for the clinical goal of patient safety	D
F	Failure mode and effects analysis with team member involvement	D
E	Environment and equipment to support patient safety	D

Grade of evidence: A, from well-designed meta-analysis; B, from well-designed controlled trials, both randomized and nonrandomized, with results that consistently support a specific action; C, from observational studies; D, from expert opinion or multiple case reports.

Adherence to established policies and procedures

Long and Johnson [55] found that adherence to established policies and procedures of medication administration was poor and that 72% of medication errors were attributed to the failure of the staff to follow policies. Evidence-based policies, guidelines, and protocols encourage communication among the disciplines and reduce medication errors. Examples include ensuring that the patient's body weight is obtained, that automatic stop orders are complied with, and that standing orders are individualized [56]. Conclusions from Cooper's study [24] suggest that the lack of adherence to policies may be due to a lack of a practical policy, and he recommends that all staff who participate in medication-related activities should be involved in the development of policies.

Policies and procedures need to be regularly updated to ensure consistency with the current evidence-based best practice. Some recommended practice changes for incorporation into policies and procedures are summarized in Box 1. Also, the Institute for Safe Medication Practices has published a list of abbreviations, symbols, and dose designations that have contributed to medication errors, available at http://www.ismp.org/PDF/ISMPAbbreviations.pdf.

Technology

In a survey of senior-level executives, department heads, and managers conducted by the Health care Information and Management Systems Society, 93% of respondents identified medication errors as a patient safety issue that technology can address [57]. The use of technology in the form of robots used for filling prescriptions, automated dispensing devices, automated medication administration record, computerized provider order entry (CPOE), "smart" intravenous devices, and barcode-enabled point-of-care (BPOC) systems are all advocated technological methods for prevention of medication errors [58,59]. These technologies can effect a significant reduction in medication errors.

With CPOE, the prescribing provider personally enters the prescription into the computer, and then the prescription is transmitted to the pharmacy. Legibility, accuracy, and avoidance of transcription errors are all key advantages. This technology can also force decisions to ensure completeness and accuracy of prescriptions. A recent study showed that CPOE could reduce medication errors by 55% or more [60].

BPOC enables nurses to use computerized databases to verify the five rights (ie, the right drug in the right dose by the right route of administration to the right patient at the right time). The process is initiated when all hospital patients are given a barcoded wristband. When a nurse scans his/her own name tag and then the patient's wristband with a hand-held device, patient information appears on a portable laptop computer, including a list of the patient's prescribed medications, drug allergies, and any other relevant health

Box 1. Recommended practice changes for incorporation into policies and procedures

- Prominently display patient allergies.
- Include the name of the drug, the dose with the unit of measurement, and the route of administration on all medication orders.
- Use generic drug nomenclature.
- Avoid trailing zeros (eg, 1.0 g), but use a zero before a decimal point (eg, 0.1mg).
- Avoid the abbreviation "u" for units (ie, spell out "units").
- Avoid abbreviations.
- Avoid verbal orders except in emergencies; if verbal orders are accepted, repeat them to the prescribing physician.
- Discontinue medication borrowing from one patient to another; eliminate any medication stashes.
- Standardize drug packaging, labeling, and storage.
- Restrict the formulary.
- Have a pharmacist review all medication orders before the first dose is administered.
- Clarify any illegible or confusing orders with the prescribing physician; do not attempt to guess what was intended.
- Double-check all calculations with another nurse or a pharmacist; have at least two ways to ensure accuracy of intravenous infusion calculations (eg, pump, manual calculation, precalculated tables).
- Use a measured weight for weight-dosed drug rather than a reported weight.
- Use premix intravenous infusion admixtures or have the infusions mixed by the pharmacist.
- Limit access to high risk drugs and use detailed protocols for the administration of these high risk drugs.
- Report all errors and near misses.

Data from Refs. [1,18,54,77,107].

information. The nurse then scans the barcode on an individual drug dose and the computer compares the scanned information against the patient's drug regimen before the drug is actually administered to the patient. An alert appears on the screen if the drug, dosage, or timing is incorrect [61,62].

Advanced BPOC technology also provides reports that reflect what errors have been made, what errors have been prevented, and a listing of reasons why nurses overrode warning messages [63]. Michael Cohen, president of the Institute for Safe Medication Practice, states "when you scan medication at the bedside, not only are you ensuring that the right medication is getting to the right patient at the right time, you are also documenting exactly what was given. Barcode systems can even tell you what wasn't given that should have been given" [62]. BPOC systems automatically provide a legible electronic copy of the medication administration record and produces reports valuable in tracking medication errors and near misses [18].

"Smart" BPOC systems provide drug reference information, alerts, and reminders [18,64]. An example of an alert would be a warning regarding look-alike or sound-alike drug names, dose exceeding maximal recommended dose, or drug allergy. A reminder would indicate important clinical actions to be taken with the drug, such as an on-screen instruction to note the patient's International Normalized Ratio before administering dicumarol (Coumadin).

The most obvious obstacle to implementing BPOC technology is that medications are not universally barcode-labeled. Currently, approximately 35% to 40% of all manufactured drugs are identified with a barcode [64,65]. However, the Food and Drug Administration has specified that a barcode will be required on the label of all drug and biological products intended for human use within 3 years [61]. Experts estimate that BPOC could decrease the medication error rate by as much as 80% [66].

Pyxis and Omnicell are examples of automated dispensing machines now found in most hospitals [67]. These unit-based medication dispensing systems communicate with the pharmacy to decrease the risk of medication error. "Smart" intravenous pumps are also available which help to prevent programming a rate that would result in a toxic drug dosage. Additional technologies are being developed that will help promote safety in drug administration.

However, system change may increase the risk for error, at least temporarily. Technologies that are intended to protect the patient may actually increase the risk of medication errors if there is inadequate preparation, education, and planning for a change process [68]. These errors may be unique, caused by staff working around the new technology and not following proper procedures. Low and Belcher [69] were surprised to find that the error rate increased by 18% in the first 24 months after implementation of BPOC (though it was not statistically significant). This increase may have been related to the automatic reporting of all discrepancies, including omissions, whereas previously the nurse was responsible for the reporting process.

Information accessibility

A study by Lesar et al [70] found that the majority of prescribing errors were caused by knowledge deficits regarding either drug therapy or patient factors that affect drug therapy. Leape's [34] research concluded that 39% of medication errors were caused by failure to disseminate drug knowledge and 18% of errors were caused by inadequate availability of patient information. The Society of Health-System Pharmacists [71] advocates the use of information that is accurate, current, comprehensive, portable, and readily accessible.

There are approximately 8000 drug products on the market today [70], which has likely contributed to the rise in medication errors. Though it is virtually impossible today to have a comprehensive working knowledge of all drugs and their effects, education regarding new drugs, restriction of the formulary, and readily available drug references may contribute to greater drug safety [56]. Although reference books are the usual resources available for nurses, these materials become outdated quickly. Personal data assistants (PDAs) such as Palm, with frequently updated software including the drug database ePocrates Rx, are extremely helpful in providing current medication information where it is needed, when it is needed, and in an easily accessible form that is current as long as updates have been downloaded. Respondents of one survey believed that the use of ePocrates Rx on a PDA prevented at least one adverse drug event per week, decreased the time required for drug selection, and increased their knowledge of medications [72]. In a survey conducted by Rothschild et al [73], physicians reported that ePocrates Rx saved time for retrieval of information, was easily incorporated into their usual work pattern, and improved drug-related decision-making. PDAs not only provide readily accessible information about drugs and calculation assistance but they can also provide clinical decision-making information at the point of patient care [74]. Internet access is also important to provide the most current drug information.

Access to complete and accurate information about the patient is also crucial. Problems in obtaining patient information include frequent difficulty in obtaining records from the patient's previous admissions, delays in documenting laboratory values that affect drug dosages (eg, serum creatinine, liver function studies) within the medical record, and slow transcription of vital signs to the paper graphic sheet. Computerized medical records allow easy access to data from previous admissions and to the most current history of the present illness. Computerized medical records are also available from remote locations with appropriate security clearance, and are therefore easily accessible to all members of the health care team.

Education regarding drug safety

Education regarding medication therapy has traditionally been focused on rituals, such as the five rights. However, Wolf [10] believes that the five rights can give a false sense of security. For instance, errors of omission would not violate any of the five rights, but if a patient does not get his medication, this would certainly be considered a medication error. Pepper

[75] writes that the five rights approach does not encourage clinical judgment by the nurse and others believe that these five rights do not take into account the significance of human factors in errors [76].

Suggested content for staff education includes information on new medications; high-alert drugs which have been identified as having the greatest potential for patient harm if an error occurs; drugs with unusual dosing considerations; policies, procedures, and protocols related to drug therapy; and strategies to prevent medication errors [77]. Leape [34] recommends training with emphasis on problem solving and possible errors and their prevention. Furthermore, whereas most education is discipline-specific, Crane [78] recommends education within the context of the multidisciplinary team (eg, the critical care team).

The American Hospital Association advocates providing education and training programs about safety practices in their initiative "Improving Medication Safety" [79]. Education to emphasize safe drug administration adds to the clinician's knowledge regarding drugs and the process of drug delivery. In a systems approach to medication error reduction at one hospital, a 4-hour medication error prevention seminar was mandatory for all nurses and unit secretaries. This was then followed by a medication error remedial process, if indicated [80].

Pepper [75] is convinced that knowledge, rather than just the information obtained from looking up the drugs given, is needed by nurses. She writes that knowledge of pharmacology allows correlation with the disease, results of diagnostic tests, and current clinical status, and improves detection of errors, contraindications, and adverse effects.

Drug miscalculations are also a factor in medication errors. Phillips et al [81] identified that 13% of human factors are related to drug miscalculation and 14% are related to a knowledge deficit. Bindler and Bayne [82] found that in a study involving 110 registered nurses, 81% were unable to calculate medication doses at a 90% pass level on a 20-item medication calculation test. In another study examining the incidence and nature of medication errors, 91% of the errors were conceptual (eg, difficulty setting up the problem) rather than arithmetic (eg, incorrect addition, subtraction, multiplication, division, or use of decimals and fractions) [83]. O'Shea [84] advocates emphasis being placed on conceptual problem solving.

Hospitals frequently require annual pharmacology tests that include questions about drugs and drug administration. Ludwig-Beymer et al [85] found that there was no change in the rate of medication error after elimination of such an annual examination.

Nonpunitive approach

A culture that blames individuals drives errors underground and results in a loss of opportunities to improve the system. Leape [34] believes that only when errors are accepted as an inevitable part of everyday practice will it be possible for hospital personnel to shift attitudes from the traditional punitive to the creative, which looks for and identifies the underlying system failures. He believes that errors should not be recorded as someone's fault, as if caused by lack of sufficient attention or caring. Although the proximal error leading to an accident is usually human error, the causes of the error are often beyond the individual's control. Leape emphasizes that all humans err frequently and that systems that rely on error-free performance are destined to fail.

Teamwork: communication and collaboration

Teamwork is essential to a safe, effective medication delivery system [71]. Teams are effective when members monitor each other's performance and provide assistance when needed, give and receive feedback, and ensure effective communication with senders by checking that the message was received as intended [86]. Team-building activities should be encouraged during the development of a culture of safety.

Benner [87] writes that the competence of individuals does not ensure competent team performance. Open discussion of differences enhances teamwork and a safer atmosphere. Every team member should be encouraged to identify potential errors before they occur and to ask questions if something does not seem right [88]. A collaborative culture is characterized by mutual respect and is one where diverse perspectives are welcomed [71]. Because an error is usually the result of a chain of events, team members who work together, have respectful conversations, and cross-monitor each other have a better chance of intercepting an error before it causes patient injury [87].

Recognition of the contribution of each team member is important in developing a team that values and protects patient safety. Members of the health care team must know their own role and understand the roles of other members.

Errors made in the ordering phase are intercepted 48% to 70% of the time because there are subsequent opportunities for validation once the orders have been charted [6,17]. An excellent example of how a multidisciplinary team provides this human safety net was identified by Leape et al [89], who found that pharmacist participation during patient rounds decreased the rate of preventable prescription ADEs by 66% and that pharmacists' recommendations regarding drug ordering were accepted by the physician 99% of the time. The human safety net requires all team members to be diligent and active participants in decision-making and to respect the contribution of other team members.

Staffing

Staffing is one of the latent system failures receiving significant attention in light of the current nursing shortage. In a study by Blendon et al [90], nurse understaffing was ranked by the public and physicians as one of the greatest threats to patient safety. "Understaffing of nurses in hospitals" and "overwork, stress, or fatigue on the part of health professionals" were cited by more than half of the physicians surveyed as key causes of medication errors. Considering the fact that nurses spend up to 40% of their time administering drugs [91], the concern is warranted.

Over the last decade, many research studies have found a link between registered nurse staffing and quality of care indicators. In 2002, a study by Aiken and colleagues [92] revealed that in hospitals with high patient–to–nurse ratios, there are higher risk-adjusted 30-day mortality and failure-to-rescue rates among surgical patients. Kovner and Gergen [93] found an inverse relationship between nurse staffing and adverse events, such as urinary tract infection and pneumonia. Unruh [94] found a greater incidence of nearly all adverse events in hospitals with fewer licensed nurses. Whitman et al [95] found an inverse relationship between staffing and falls in cardiac intensive care, medication errors in both cardiac and noncardiac intensive care units, and restraint rates in the medical-surgical units. Sasichay-Akkadechanunt and colleagues [96] found that the ratio of total nurse staffing was significantly related to inpatient mortality, but did not find a relationship between mortality and skill mix, experience, or educational level.

Nurses perceive lack of knowledge and experience as factors that contribute to medication errors [97]. In addition to formal education, experiential learning has been shown to decrease medication errors. In a study intended to reveal the relationship between the quality of patient care and the education and experience of the nurses providing the care, units with more experienced nurses had lower medication error rates, although formal education (eg, BSN) did not significantly reduce medication errors [98]. However, Aiken et al [99] found that surgical patients in hospitals that had a higher proportion of registered nurses with bachelor's degrees who were administering direct care had a lower mortality rate than patients treated in hospitals that had fewer nurses with bachelor's degrees.

Blegen et al [98] found that the higher the RN skill mix, the lower the incidence of adverse occurrences (including medication errors) on inpatient care units. Needleman and colleagues [100] also found a lower incidence of adverse occurrences where a higher RN skill mix existed, but did not include medication errors as one of the adverse effects (included were pneumonia, upper gastrointestinal bleeding, shock, sepsis, and deep vein thrombosis).

Staffing ratios have received national attention. California has already established mandatory staffing ratios. Pronovost et al [101] found that in hospitals where the critical care nurse–to–patient ratio was one nurse to three or more patients, there was an increased risk for several specific pulmonary complications (eg, pulmonary insufficiency, reintubation), as opposed to hospitals with ratios in the critical care units of one nurse to one or two patients.

Patient assignments should match the complexity of the condition to the competencies of the nurse [102]. For instance, the expert nurse should be assigned to the highest acuity patient. Efforts should also be made to match specific proficiencies of the nurse to the specific needs of the patient.

Administrative support for the clinical goal of patient safety

Organizational leadership, including governing boards, administration, and clinical leadership must be committed to safety [45,103]. Activities that communicate this commitment include addressing safety in the strategic plans of the organization and on the board meeting agendas; having policies and procedures that address responsibilities regarding patient safety; establishing safety goals and monitoring of achievement of these goals; and budgeting and appropriating direct resources for patient safety programs [45]. All employees need to be empowered and vigilant to patient's needs for safety. Key aspects of this empowerment are communication, nonhierarchical decision making, training, and rewards and incentives for involvement and innovation in safety improvements [45]. Employees should be encouraged to identify potential unsafe situations and possibilities for error before errors actually occur [88]. Administrators should promote a questioning environment among their staff.

Failure mode and effects analysis with team member involvement

A failure mode and effects analysis is a process previously adopted by other industries, such as aviation and automobile manufacturing, in which a system is analyzed to determine potential problems and how to avoid them. This analysis anticipates Murphy's Law (ie, whatever can happen will happen) and aims to prevent system failures before they occur [104]. The goal is to detect errors, alert staff, eliminate the possibilities of intolerable errors, and prevent the error before it occurs, or, at the very least, minimize the consequences of the error [105]. A flow chart of the process is developed and potential latent errors are identified; the potential impact and probability of the error is anticipated; and plans are developed to decrease the chance of error [56].

Cohen identifies four basic aspects of error prevention, including: (1) removal of (undesirable) alternatives, (2) improvement in detection, (3) prevention of (incorrect) action completion, and (4) minimization of the consequence of the error [104]. Attention to these points would be particularly helpful during a failure mode analysis of the drug administration processes at an institution.

Environment and equipment

Environmental factors can significantly affect the risk for errors. Adequate lighting is required for preparing and administering medications. An area that is free of distraction and excessive noise allows for concentration when providers are calculating, preparing, and administering medications. Therefore, separate physical facilities for preparing and administering medications are recommended. Facilities for handwashing must be available and convenient.

Elimination of infusion pumps without free-flow protection was one of the 2003 national patient safety goals released by the Joint Commission on Accreditation of Healthcare Organizations [106]. Use of appropriate equipment for a given situation must be ensured. For example, standard intravenous tubing with injection ports should not be used for continuous enteral feedings because medication errors have occurred when the nurse injected an antacid into intravenous tubing that was thought to be the continuous enteral feeding tubing. Supplies needed for the administration of medications (eg, syringes, pumps, filters, and labels) need to be available and conveniently located. Patient-controlled analgesia and epidural analgesia pumps need to be easily programmable and reliable. The initiation of CPOE and BPOC requires major capital expenditures for hardware and software, but the proven benefits to reducing medication errors substantiates these expenditures.

Summary

Medication errors are costly from human, economic, and societal perspectives. All patients are vulnerable to the detrimental effects of these errors. Recommendations regarding the problem of medication errors include:

- Prevention of error by learning from the nonpunitive reporting of errors and near misses
- Evaluation of the system for potential causes of error through failure mode and effects analysis and encouragement of a questioning attitude
- Elimination of system problems that increase the risk of error
- Recognition that humans are fallible and that error will occur even in a perfect system
- Minimization of the consequences of errors when they do occur

An important goal for healthcare organizations should be to create a culture that accepts the imperfection of human performance and solicits the assistance of team members in the development of safeguards for error prevention. Proposed interventions to prevent medication errors can be described by the PATIENT SAFE taxonomy, which includes:

- Patient participation
- Adherence to established policy and procedures
- Technology use
- Information accessibility
- Education regarding medication safety
- Nonpunitive approach to reporting of errors and near misses

- Teamwork, communication, and collaboration
- Staffing: adequate number and staffing mix
- Administration support for the clinical goal of patient safety
- Failure mode and effects analysis with team member involvement
- Environment and equipment to support patient safety

References

[1] Kohn LT, Corrigan JM, Donaldson MS, editors. To err is human: building a safer health system. Washington, DC: National Academy Press; 1999.
[2] Bridge Medical. Timeline for medication error prevention. Available at: www.mederrors.com/resource_main_set.html. Accessed November 15, 2002.
[3] Leape LL, Brennan TA, Laird N, et al. The nature of adverse events in hospitalized patients. Results of the Harvard Medical Practice Study II. N Engl J Med 1991;324:377–84.
[4] American Society of Health-System Pharmacists. Suggested definitions and relationships among medication misadventures, medication errors, adverse drug events, and adverse drug reactions. Am J Health Syst Pharm 1998;55:165–6.
[5] Bates DW, Boyle DL, Vander Vliet MB, et al. Relationship between medication errors and adverse drug events. J Gen Intern Med 1995;10:199–205.
[6] Bates DW, Cullen DJ, Laird N, et al. Incidence of adverse drug effects and potential adverse drug effects. Implications for prevention. JAMA 1995;274(1):29–34.
[7] Bates DW, Leape LL, Petrycki S. Incidence and preventability of adverse drug events in hospitalized adults. J Gen Intern Med 1993;8:289–94.
[8] Bates DW. Medication errors. How common are they and what can be done to prevent them? Drug Saf 1996;15:303–10.
[9] Bond CA, Raehl C, Franke T. Medication errors in United States hospitals. Pharmacotherapy 2001;21(9):1023–36.
[10] Wolf ZR. Medication errors and nursing responsibility. Holist Nurs Pract 1989;4(1):8–17.
[11] Serembus JF, Wolf ZR, Youngblood N. Consequences of fatal medication errors for health care providers: A secondary analysis study. Medsurg Nurs 2001;10(4):193–201.
[12] Bates DW, Spell N, Cullen DJ, et al. The costs of adverse drug events in hospitalized patients. JAMA 1997;277(4):307–11.
[13] Classen DC, Pestotnik SL, Evans RS, et al. Adverse drug events in hospitalized patients. Excess length of stay, extra costs, and attributable mortality. JAMA 1997;277(4):301–6.
[14] Johnson JA, Bootman JL. Drug-related morbidity and mortality. A cost-of-illness model. Arch Intern Med 1995;155:1949–56.
[15] Lewin-VHI. Nursing report card for acute care settings. Washington, DC: American Nurses Publishing; 1995.
[16] Scholz DA. Establishing and monitoring an endemic medication error rate. J Nurs Qual Assur 1990;4(2):71–85.
[17] Leape LL. System analysis of adverse drug events. JAMA 1995;274(1):25–43.
[18] Brown MM. Managing medication errors by design. Crit Care Nurs Q 2001;24(3):77–97.
[19] Olsen K. Medication errors: problems identified, but what is the solution? Crit Care Med 2002;30(4):944–5.
[20] Weingart S, Wilson R, Gibberd R, et al. Epidemiology of medical error. BMJ 2000;320:774–7.
[21] Wilson RM, Runciman WB, Gibberd RW, et al. The Quality in Australian Health Care Study. Med J Aust 1995;163:458–71.
[22] Chassin MR. Is health care ready for Six Sigma quality? Milbank Q 1998;76(4):565–91.
[23] Lanham B, Maxson-Cooper P. Is Six Sigma the answer for nursing to reduce medical errors and enhance patient safety? Nurs Econ 2003;21(1):39–41.

[24] Cooper M. Can a zero defects philosophy be applied to drug errors? J Adv Nurs 1995;21(3): 487–91.

[25] Anderson D, Webster CS. A systems approach to the approach of medication error on the hospital ward. J Adv Nurs 2001;35(1):34–41.

[26] Larrabee JH, Ruckstuhl M, Salmons J, et al. Interdisciplinary monitoring of medication errors in a nursing quality assurance program. Nursing Quality Assurance 1991;5(4):69–78.

[27] Greene J. From whodunit to what happened. Hosp Health Netw 1999;73(4):50–4.

[28] Osborne J, Blais K, Hayes J. Nurses' perceptions: when is it a medication error? J Nurs Adm 1999;29(4):33–8.

[29] Gladstone J. Drug administration errors: a study into the factors underlying the occurrence and reporting of drug errors in a district general hospital. J Adv Nurs 1995;22(4):628–37.

[30] Murphy MD. Individual characteristics of nurses who committed medication administration errors. Cases which resulted in licensure discipline by the Colorado Board of Nursing. Issues 1992;13:11–3.

[31] Cohen H, Robinson ES, Mandrack M. Getting to the root of medication errors: survey results. Nursing 2003;33(9):36–46.

[32] Crane VS. New perspectives on preventing medication errors and adverse drug events. Am J Health Syst Pharm 2000;57(7):690–7.

[33] Rasmussen J, Jensen A. Mental procedures in real-life tasks: a case study of electronic trouble shooting. Ergonomics 1974;17:293–307.

[34] Leape LL. Error in medicine. JAMA 1994;272(23):1851–7.

[35] Kelly WN. Potential risks and prevention, part 4: reports of significant drug errors. Am J Health Syst Pharm 2001;58(15):1406–12.

[36] Reason J. Human error. Cambridge (England): Cambridge University Press; 1990.

[37] Reason J. Understanding adverse events: human factors. In: Vincent C, editor. Clinical risk management. London: BMJ Publishing Group; 1995. p. 31–54.

[38] Meurier CE. Understanding the nature of errors in nursing: using a model to analyse critical incident reports of errors which had resulted in an adverse or potentially adverse event. J Adv Nurs 2000;32(1):202–7.

[39] Reason J. Human error: models and management. BMJ 2000;320:768–70.

[40] Pronovost P, Wu AW, Dorman T, et al. Building safety into ICU care. J Crit Care 2002; 17(2):78–85.

[41] Crow SM, Hartman SJ. Organizational culture: its impact on employee relations and discipline in health care organizations. Health Care Manag (Frederick) 2002;21(2):22–8.

[42] Carson S. Organisational Change. In: Hamer S, Collinson G, editors. Achieving evidence-based practice: a handbook for practitioners. Leeds (UK): Bailliere Tindall; 1999.

[43] Closs SJ, Cheater FM. Utilization of nursing research: culture, interest, and support. J Adv Nurs 1994;19:762–73.

[44] Cooper M. Towards a model of safety culture. Safety Science 2000;36:111–36.

[45] Page A, editor. Keeping patients safe: transforming the work environment for nurses. Washington, DC: National Academy Press; 2003.

[46] Killen AR, Beyea SC. Learning from near misses in an effort to promote patient safety. AORN J 2003;77(2):423–5.

[47] Tokarski C. Effective practices: Improve Patient Safety Summit 2001. Medscape Managed Care 2001;1(1):1009.

[48] Wakefield BJ, Wakefield DS, Uden-Holman T, et al. Nurses' perceptions of why medication administration errors occur. Medsurg Nurs 1998;7(1):39–43.

[49] Sutton J, Standen P, Wallace A. Incidence and documentation of patient accidents in hospital. Nurs Times 1994;90(33):29–35.

[50] Hackel R, Butt L, Banister G. How nurses perceive medication errors. Nurs Manage 1996; 27(1):33–4.

[51] Elnitsky C, Nichols B, Palmer K. Are hospital incidents being reported? J Nurs Adm 1997; 27(11):40–6.

[52] Agency for Healthcare Research and Quality. Medical errors: the scope of the problem. An epidemic of errors. Available at: www.ahrq.gov/qual/errback.htm. Accessed December 4, 2001.

[53] Aspden P, Corrigan JM, Wolcott J, et al, editors. Patient safety: achieving a new standard for care. Washington, DC: National Academy Press; 2004.

[54] Carroll P. Medication errors. The bigger picture. RN 2003;66(1):52–8.

[55] Long G, Johnson C. A pilot study for reducing medication errors. QRB Qual Rev Bull 1981;7(4):6–9.

[56] Lindquist R, Gersema L. Understanding and preventing adverse drug effects. AACN Clin Issues 1998;9(1):119–28.

[57] Healthcare Information Management System Society. Patient Safety Survey HIMSS. Available at: www.infosolutions.mckesson.com/himsspatient/survey.asp. Accessed December 9, 2003.

[58] Bates DW. Using information technology to reduce rates of medication errors in hospitals. BMJ 2000;320:788–91.

[59] Kaushal R, Shojania KG, Bates DW. Effects of computerized physician order entry and clinical decision support systems on medication safety. Arch Intern Med 2003;163(12): 1409–16.

[60] Bates DW, Leape LL, Cullen DJ, et al. Effect of computerized physician order entry and a team intervention on prevention of serious medication errors. JAMA 1998;280(15): 1311–6.

[61] US Food Drug Administration. Questions and answers regarding the bar code proposal. Available at: www.fda.gov/oc/initiatives/barcode-sadr/qa-barcode.html. Accessed December 7, 2003.

[62] Wiebe C. Patient safety concerns could spur bar code adoption. Medscape Money & Medicine 2002;3(2):1–3.

[63] Douglas J, Larrabee S. Bring barcoding to the bedside. Nurs Manage 2003;34(5):36–40.

[64] Medpathways. Pathways for medication safety: assessing bedside bar-coding readiness. Available at: www.medpathways.info. Accessed December 9, 2003.

[65] Sublett P. Reducing medication errors through technology and process change. In: Healthcare Information and Management Systems Society 2003. Available at: http:// www.himss.org/content/files/proceedings/2003/Sessions/session131.pdf.

[66] Haugh R. Bar code bandwagon. Hosp Health Netw 2003;77(5):55–6.

[67] Posey LM. Medication errors: technology coming to the rescue. Pharmacy Today 2002; 8(2):1, 11.

[68] Yan J. The human factor in medication-error reduction. Am J Health Syst Pharm 2003;60: 1417.

[69] Low DK, Belcher JV. Reporting medication errors through computerized medication administration. CIN. Comput Inform Nurs 2002;20(5):178–83.

[70] Lesar TS, Briceland L, Stein DS. Factors related to errors in medication prescribing. JAMA 1997;277(4):312–7.

[71] Pharmacy-nursing shared vision for safe medication use in hospitals: executive session summary. Am J Health Syst Pharm 2003;60:1046–52.

[72] Rempher KJ, Lasome CE, Lasome TJ. Leveraging palm technology in the advanced practice nursing environment. AACN Clin Issues 2003;14(3):363–70.

[73] Rothschild JM, Lee TH, Bae T, Bates DW. Clinician use of a palmtop drug reference guide. J Am Med Inform Assoc 2002;9(3):223–9.

[74] Galt KA, Rich EC, Young WW. Impact of hand-held technologies on medication errors in primary care. Top Health Inf Manage 2002;23(2):71–81.

[75] Pepper GA. Errors in drug administration by nurses. Am J Health Syst Pharm 1995;52: 390–5.

[76] Institute for Safe Medication Practices. The "five rights." Available at: www.ismp.org/ MSAarticles/FiveRights.htm. Accessed December 4, 2001.

[77] Smetzer J. Take 10 giant steps to medication safety. Nursing 2001;31(11):49–54.

[78] Crane VS. New perspectives on preventing medication errors and adverse drug events. Am J Health Syst Pharm 2000;57:690–7.

[79] American Hospital Association. AHA initiative: improving medication safety. Available at: www.aha.org/medicationsafety/AHAinitiative.asp. Accessed December 4, 2001.

[80] Schaubhut R, Jones C. A systems approach to medication error reduction. J Nurs Care Qual 2000;14(3):13–27.

[81] Phillips J, Beam S, Brinker A, et al. Retrospective analysis of mortalities associated with medication errors. Am J Health Syst Pharm 2001;58(19):1824–9.

[82] Bindler R, Bayne T. Medication calculation ability of registered nurses. Image J Nurs Sch 1991;23(4):221–4.

[83] Segatore M, Edge D, Miller M. Posology errors by sophomore nursing students. Nurs Outlook 1993;41(4):160–5.

[84] O'Shea E. Factors contributing to medication errors: a literature review. J Clin Nurs 1999; 8(5):496–504.

[85] Ludwig-Beymer P, Czurylo KT, Gattuso MC, et al. The effect of testing on the reported incidence of medication errors in a medical center. J Contin Educ Nurs 1990;21(1):11–7.

[86] Firth-Cozens J. Cultures for improving patient safety through learning: the role of teamwork. Qual Health Care 2001;10(4):26–31.

[87] Benner P. Creating a culture of safety and improvement: a key to reducing medical error. Am J Crit Care 2001;10(4):281–4.

[88] Watson D. Creating the culture of safety. AORN J 2003;77(2):268–71.

[89] Leape LL, Cullen DJ, Clapp MD, et al. Pharmacist participation on physician rounds and adverse drug events in the intensive care unit. JAMA 1999;282(3):267–70.

[90] Blendon RJ, DesRoches CM, Brodie M, et al. Views of practicing physicians and the public on medical errors. N Engl J Med 2002;347(24):1933–40.

[91] Armitage G, Knapman H. Adverse events in drug administration: a literature review. J Nurs Manag 2003;11:130–40.

[92] Aiken LH, Clarke SP, Sloane DM, et al. Hospital nurse staffing and patient mortality, nurse burnout, and job dissatisfaction. JAMA 2002;288(16):1987–93.

[93] Kovner C, Gergen PJ. Nurse staffing levels and adverse events following surgery in U.S. Hospitals. Image J Nurs Sch 1998;30:315–21.

[94] Unruh L. Licensed nurse staffing and adverse events in hospitals. Med Care 2003;41(1): 142–52.

[95] Whitman GR, Kim Y, Davidson LJ, et al. The impact of staffing on patient outcomes across specialty units. J Nurs Adm 2002;32(12):633–9.

[96] Sasichay-Akkadechanunt T, Scalzi CG, Jawad AF. The relationship between nurse staffing and patient outcomes. J Nurs Adm 2003;33(9):478–85.

[97] Meurier CE, Vincent CA, Parmar DG. Learning from errors in nursing practice. J Adv Nurs 1997;26(1):111–9.

[98] Blegen MA, Goode CJ, Reed L. Nurse staffing and patient outcomes. Nurs Res 1998;47(1): 43–50.

[99] Aiken LH, Clarke SP, Cheung RB, et al. Educational levels of hospital nurses and surgical patient mortality. JAMA 2003;290(12):1617–23.

[100] Needleman J, Buerhaus P, Mattke S, et al. Nurse-staffing levels and the quality of care in hospitals. N Engl J Med 2002;346(22):1715–22.

[101] Pronovost PJ, Dang D, Dorman T, et al. Intensive care unit nurse staffing and the risk for complications after abdominal aortic surgery. Eff Clin Pract 2001;4:223–5.

[102] Curley MA. Patient-nurse synergy: optimizing patients' outcomes. Am J Crit Care 1998; 7(1):64–72.

[103] Spath PL. Does your facility have a "patient-safe" climate? Hosp Peer Rev 2000;25:80–2.

[104] Cohen MR, Senders J, Davis NM. Failure mode and effects analysis: a novel approach to avoiding dangerous medication errors and accidents. Hosp Pharm 1994;29:319–28.

[105] Fletcher C. Failure mode and effects analysis. An interdisciplinary way to analyze and reduce medication errors. J Nurs Adm 1997;27(12):19–26.

[106] Joint Commission on Accreditation of Healthcare Organizations. 2003 National Patient Safety Goals. Available at: http://www.jcaho.org/accredited + organizations/patient + safety/04 + npsg/04_npsg.htm. Accessed December 28, 2003.

[107] Summerfield MR, Lawence T. Rethinking approaches to reducing medication errors: an examination of 10 core processes. Formulary 2002;37(9):462.

ELSEVIER
SAUNDERS

NURSING
CLINICS
OF NORTH AMERICA

Nurs Clin N Am 40 (2005) 25–32

Reduction of Adverse Drug Events and Medication Errors in a Community Hospital Setting

Deborah S. Smith, RN, MS, MBA, CNAA*,
Kathy Haig, RN

OSF St. Joseph Medical Center, 2200 E. Washington, Bloomington, IL 61701, USA

According to the Institute of Medicine's 1999 report *To Err is Human: Building a Safer Health System* [1], between 44,000 and 98,000 people die annually in United States hospitals as a result of preventable medical errors. The same report estimates the yearly cost of these errors to be approximately $29 billion.

Medication errors are preventable mistakes that often occur when drugs are prescribed or administered erroneously or incorrectly to patients, frequently causing harm [2]. An adverse drug event (ADE) is "an excessive response to a medication that is undesired or unexpected" [3]. Bates et al [4] published a case control study in 1997 demonstrating that average hospital lengths of stay increased by 2.2 days and accrued an associated cost of $3244 for patients who experienced an ADE. For a 700-bed teaching hospital, this amounted to an annual cost of $5.6 million.

Because multiple clinicians are involved in the process of prescribing and administering medication, medication errors are a multidisciplinary problem [5]. Therefore, the use of a multidisciplinary team is essential in identifying and implementing measures for improvement.

Medline and CINAHL database searches for the phrase "patient safety" obtained over 5300 results (February 2004). A Google internet search yielded over 3.8 million "hits" for the same subject. Newspapers, magazines, government agency reports, insurers, and accrediting bodies have all picked up the banner of patient safety and are flying it high.

* Corresponding author.
 E-mail address: debsdarb@msn.com (D.S. Smith).

This discussion does not describe a comprehensive patient safety initiative but instead focuses on one hospital's experience in reducing medication errors and ADEs and improving the safety of its patients.

St. Joseph Medical Center (SJMC) is one of six acute care hospitals owned and operated by the Sisters of the Third Order of Saint Francis (OSF) Healthcare System. The hospital is licensed for 180 beds and is a non-profit facility that serves a community of 110,000 in central Illinois. The facility provides a full array of inpatient and outpatient services including invasive cardiology and neurology, cardiovascular surgery and neurosurgery, and a Level II Trauma Center. SJMC also operates an urgent care center, five physician office practices, and several outpatient joint ventures with physician partners. SJMC provides 24-hour pharmacy services and has recently deployed clinical pharmacists to inpatient units on a daily basis.

Early attempts

To measure ADEs, one must be aware of when these events occur. Initially, the only notifications the SJMC administration received were incident occurrence reports. Leadership and risk management personnel suspected this was only the "tip of the iceberg" regarding actual events. The clinical staff's fear of disciplinary action or counseling and their distaste for the required, cumbersome paperwork likely reduced the reporting of errors. Early in 2000, SJMC adopted and promoted a new reporting policy that encourages staff to report adverse events without fear of reprisal. Orientation sessions and annual workshops provide ongoing education emphasizing the importance of reporting ADEs. Two primary reasons for reporting are to enable immediate and appropriate care to be provided to the patient, and to initiate evaluation of the incident to reduce future potential for error. The prevailing belief is that errors are unintentional, caused by poor systems or processes, and complicated by human factors.

An ADE hotline was also established at SJMC in early 2000, providing a site where any error or adverse event made or discovered can be reported. Details including the date of the event, patient name, medication involved, and the nature of the event are recorded on a well-publicized hospital extension. A pharmacist checks the hotline daily, initiates investigation into the events and potential causes, and completes the incident occurrence report. Use of the hotline does not eliminate the need to notify physicians and to intervene regarding errors, but facilitates the reporting of errors.

The hotline provides a mechanism for staff to anonymously report a medication event. This is a "win–win" situation because the staff can report the event easily, anonymously, and quickly by avoiding the usual paperwork, and the event can also be identified for evaluation and trending.

Methodology–a collaborative approach

Changing the culture

Culture is defined as "the set of shared attitudes, values, goals, and practices that characterizes a company or corporation" [6]. With this in mind, SJMC initiated a comprehensive redesign of its culture and care systems in an effort to reduce the potential rate of harm to patients. Reduction of events involving medications was identified as the area in need of improvement that impacted the largest population of patients. Flowcharting revealed medication processes to be complicated and labor intensive, and to involve multiple caregivers from the time the order is written until the patient receives the medication. Common sources of errors included:

- Unavailable patient information
- Unavailable drug information
- Miscommunication of medication orders
- Problems with labeling or packaging
- Drug standardization
- Improper storage
- Incorrect stocking of inventory
- Process flaws

To facilitate this culture- and system-improvement project, SJMC entered into a collaborative with the Institute of Healthcare Improvement (IHI) as one of 50 international hospitals to participate in a program addressing the reduction of ADEs. The program's leadership provided both human and financial resources and a team of early-adopters was established representing nursing, administration, medical, and pharmacy staff. This core group was sent to three 2-day training sessions provided by the IHI. Aims and goals were established, including (1) maintenance of a specific cultural survey score, (2) use of the medication reconciliation process, (3) reduction in the Dispensing Failure Mode Effects Analysis (FMEA), and (3) reduction of events occurring with high-risk medications.

To promote patient safety throughout the environment, safety must become a priority in the organization's culture. SJMC conducted cultural surveys every 6 months to determine the willingness of staff to report adverse events. The survey was obtained from the IHI and is a modified version of the Brian Sexton/Robert Helmreich aviation cultural survey [7]. Respondents included 10% each of hospital and medical staff. The survey lists nine statements and uses a Likert-type scale ranging from one to five to indicate agreement or disagreement. The survey was used as a tool to measure the effectiveness of promoting a nonpunitive culture to report safety concerns. Survey results in the first year improved from a 3.96 baseline score to 4.28, with 5.0 as the maximum score possible.

One of the lessons learned from the survey is that changing the culture of an institution is a very slow process. SJMC is currently evaluating a new survey tool that addresses teamwork concepts in addition to attitudes regarding the safety culture of the organization, and these will be conducted annually.

To involve the physicians in the culture of safety, patient safety has been added as a standing agenda item in all medical staff quality meetings. Feedback regarding safety concerns identified in safety briefings, and results of any root cause analysis of near misses are also shared with medical staff in their quality-management meetings.

Root cause analysis of near misses includes input from all staff directly involved, including nurses, allied health care providers, and physicians. In response to the belief that events are the cause of poor processes, human factor components including communication, environment, staffing, equipment, and competency have been incorporated into the review process. This has been instrumental in trying to eliminate blame.

Reconciliation

A key tool used by SJMC in the reduction of ADEs is the medication reconciliation process. Medication reconciliation is a tool used to convey information regarding patient medication at the various points where such information is passed along [8]. Medication reconciliation is the act of comparing the medications the patient has been taking with the medications currently ordered. This allows the caregiver to identify medications that may need to be continued, discontinued, or that require dose or frequency adjustments based on the patient's changing condition. The comparison is conducted during three phases: admission, transfer, and discharge. On admission reconciliation, the home medications are compared with the initial physician orders. On transfer reconciliation, the medications the patient was taking in the previous nursing unit are compared to the orders in the current unit. And on discharge reconciliation, the list of medications taken while in the hospital is compared with the list of medications ordered for the patient upon discharge. The nurse or pharmacist should reconcile any variations between the two lists with the physician within 4 or 24 hours, depending on the type of medication. Because a physician signature line is present, the medication discharge order sheet can also save time and potential transcription errors by serving as the medication order sheet.

SJMC achieved accurate admission reconciliation ranges of 85% to 95%, an accurate transfer reconciliation of 70%, and an accurate discharge reconciliation of 95%, prior to the implementation of an electronic medical record system.

The implementation of the new medical record process caused a brief decline in reconciliation rates, but these are again beginning to show improvement. However, there appears to be a direct correlation between use of the reconciliation process and the ADE rate, as evidenced by the slight increase in the number of ADEs immediately following implementation of the computerized medical record system, when the use of the reconciliation process briefly declined. (Fig. 1).

Failure mode event analysis

SJMC's dispensing Failure Mode and Effect Analysis (FMEA) score has dropped 66% in the past 2 years as a result of multiple action steps. The FMEA identifies the various ways a process may fail [9]. As a result of the analysis, the retrieval of discharged patients' medications from the medication cart on each nursing unit was changed from every 24 hours to hourly. Additionally, stock medications on the patient care units have been reduced by 45%, adult intravenous (IV) medications have been standardized, and all nonstandard doses are prepared by the pharmacy. An IV drug administration reference matrix directing dosage, guidelines, and monitoring information has been developed for nursing staff. A pharmacist compares lab values with orders to identify potentially inappropriate dosing. Anesthesia staff have contributed to the reduction of potential dispensing events by assisting in standardization of epidural-safe pumps using colored tubing.

Standardized order sets

As standardization of orders is believed to be an important factor in reducing variance, pharmacy-based services and order sets have aided efforts in the reduction of ADEs. Both inpatient and outpatient warfarin dosing service is offered by the pharmacy. A patient controlled analgesia order set was developed and has achieved a usage rate of 93%. This order set offers default doses on selected medications for pain management. A total parenteral nutrition order set and dosing service is now used at a rate of 100% and renal dosing services are also conducted for all patients having a creatinine clearance of less than 50 mL.

One of the most popular changes SJMC made was the staffing of pharmacists on the patient care units to review and enter medication orders. This provided the double benefit of saving nursing time and providing the pharmacist a first-hand look at the orders, thereby allowing the identification of potential dosing errors and drug interactions. Because of these efforts, a 34% improvement was noted in the ordering FMEA hazard vulnerability score, decreasing it from 157 to 103.

High-risk medications

To address high-risk medications, SJMC made a focused effort to eliminate the multiple order sets for heparin use within the organization. An interdisciplinary team of nurses, pharmacists, and physicians developed an

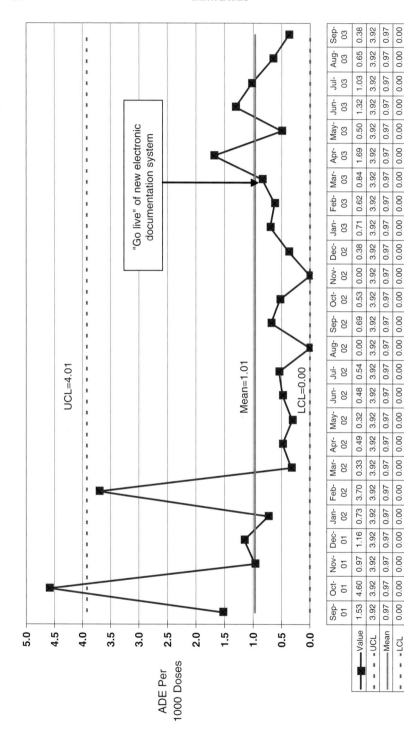

[Sep-01 To Present : IHI-ADE Data]

evidence-based order set and conducted rapid cycle tests of change, at which point the order set was adopted throughout the organization. Other high-risk medication protocols are currently in various stages of development, including sedation and IV insulin protocols.

Additional tools

The availability of a simulation laboratory at SJMC provides the ability to recreate quality concerns, investigate process failures, complete a Root Cause Analysis, and identify failure modes. The laboratory imitates a hospital setting and includes video equipment to tape the simulation for the debriefing process that follows every exercise. While avoiding risk to actual patients, the simulation lab allows practice in team and rapid response; evaluation of critical thinking, assessment, and technical skills; and the ability to visualize and learn from errors through the debriefing session. The manikin software allows educators to use either prepro-grammed scenarios or to program a scenario that mimics a real event. Based on the reactions of the staff in the simulation exercise, the manikin's condition can either improve or deteriorate. Simulation with the manikin is used in clinical orientation of new employees and for skills validation of current employees.

An electronic medical record system, including the medication adminis-tration record (MAR), was initiated by SJMC in March 2003. As previously stated, the change in processes did impact reconciliation scores, but the overall benefits of the EMR have been substantial. The ability to have the MAR at the patient's bedside while administering medication, and the ability for multiple clinicians to view the MAR simultaneously have been extremely beneficial.

An automated medication dispensing system became operational in November 2003, which added another level of safety to the medication administration process. Bar code verification has not been implemented as of this writing.

Summary

Keys to success in reducing ADEs have included the support of administrative leaders through their visibility and emphasis on safety as

Fig. 1. Chart revealing number of ADEs occurring per 1000 doses. There appears to be a direct correlation between use of the reconciliation process and the ADE rate, as evidenced by the slight increase in the number of ADEs immediately following implementation of the computerized medical record system, when the use of the reconciliation process briefly declined.UCL, upper control limit; LCL, lower control limit.

an organizational priority, and financial support for safety projects. Administrative participation was also helpful in promoting safety efforts through the reinforcement of expectations when progress was sluggish. The use of rapid cycle change provided enough early success to serve in motivating staff to push ahead. It allowed staff the opportunity to analyze changes, make adjustments, and retest on a slightly larger scale.

Other key success factors included the motivation of teams through continual sharing of progress and success stories; celebrations for achievements are held routinely. As an organization, SJMC has shared its success strategies with other organizations and promoted networking with other organizations to determine what strategies have worked elsewhere. This is helpful as it prevents time from being wasted on solutions that have been tried without success.

Within the OSF Healthcare System, the following phrase has been adopted in regard to patient safety, "Safety is like peeling an onion; the more you look, the more you find, and each layer makes you cry."

References

[1] Kohn LT, Corrigan JM, Donaldson MS, editors. To err is human: building a safer health system. Washington, DC: National Academy Press; 1999.
[2] Agency for Healthcare Research and Quality. Reducing errors in health care: translating research into practice. Rockville, MD: Agency for Healthcare Research and Quality; 2000. Publication No.00–PO58.
[3] Lassetter JH, Warnick ML. Medical errors, drug-related problems, and medication errors: a literature review on quality of care and cost issues. J Nurs Care Qual 2003;18(3):175–83.
[4] Bates DW, Spell N, Cullen DJ, et al. The costs of adverse drug events in hospitalized patients: adverse drug events prevention study group. JAMA 1997;277:307–11.
[5] O'Shea E. Factors contributing to medication errors: a literature review. J Clin Nurs 1999;8: 496–504.
[6] Merriam-Webster Online Dictionary. Available at: http://www.m-w.com. Accessed January 19, 2004.
[7] Sexton JB, Thomas EJ, Helmreich RL. Error, stress, and teamwork in medicine and aviation: cross sectional surveys. Br J Hosp Med 2000;320:745–9.
[8] Whittington J, Cohen H. OSF Healthcare's journey in patient safety. Q Manage Health Care 2004;13(1):53–9.
[9] Juran JM. Juran's quality control handbook. 4th edition. New York: McGraw-Hill, Inc; 1988.

ELSEVIER
SAUNDERS

NURSING
CLINICS
OF NORTH AMERICA

Nurs Clin N Am 40 (2005) 33–49

Use of Prescription Drugs: Rising or Declining?

Anita B. Crockett, PhD, RN

School of Nursing, Box 81, Middle Tennessee State University,
Murfreesboro, TN 37132, USA

In the mid-twentieth century, the United States emerged as a major drug-consumption market. Although illegal drug use and abuse received more media attention, an unprecedented increasing reliance on existing therapeutic drugs and interest in developing new drugs and drug combinations were emerging during this time. Since that time, there has been a greater acceptance of legitimate drug therapy as a solution to many of society's ills.

In 2002, health professionals were prescribing more medicines than they had in the mid-1980s. Changes in health practice account for part of the increase, particularly in health maintenance organizations where policies often encourage multiple drug use. The number of prescriptions for advertised drugs began to jump significantly in 1997 when the Food and Drug Administration (FDA) allowed direct advertising of drugs to consumers [1]. In 2001, most of the increases in drug costs occurred in four heavily advertised categories of drugs: arthritis, cholesterol, depression, and allergy [2]. A recent study shows that minority groups are particularly influenced by prescription drug ads and are more likely to believe that the government approves the ads before they are shown, which is not the case [3].

A Kaiser Family Foundation study found an association between consumer advertising expenditures and drugs that are gaining the most popularity. In response to seeing a drug advertisement, 13% of Americans have requested and received a specific prescription from their health care providers [4]. A joint Harvard–MIT study in May 2003 found that for every additional $1 spent on direct-to-consumer advertising, the pharmaceutical industry yielded an additional $4.20 in sales [5]. Although objective research is scant as to whether this type of promotion increases consumer education

---

E-mail address: acrocket@mtsu.edu

0029-6465/05/$ - see front matter © 2005 Elsevier Inc. All rights reserved.
doi:10.1016/j.cnur.2004.08.012   *nursing.theclinics.com*

or merely increases requests for the drug and the potential for inappropriate use, the upsurge in prescribing is evident.

In June 2002, President Bush authorized the third 5-year extension of the Prescription Drug User Fee Act of 1992, which expedites the FDA approval process for new drugs [6]. The number of new, approved drugs has doubled since the 1980s and the length of time for approval has shortened from an average of 33 months in 1986 to 12 months in 1998. The combination of new medications, an aging population, and new treatment patterns produced an increase of 34% in prescriptions from 1985 to 1999. The medications ordered for clients were not only those obtained through pharmacists but were also over-the-counter drugs and immunizations [7].

This increase in prescriptions has brought a concomitant increase in costs. Spending on medicines is slated to increase at about 15% per year and will double within 5 years, with no limitation for age groups. Psychiatric medications have caused the largest jump in prescriptions (attributable to antidepressants and the fact that at least eight new ones have been introduced since 1987). Six types of drug therapies are responsible for 80% of the increase: central nervous system drugs, hormones, respiratory treatments, pain relief medications, cardiovascular-renal drugs, and metabolics and nutrients. Between 1985 and 1999, prescriptions for central nervous system disorders (eg, drugs for attention-deficit hyperactivity disorder) increased 327% among children, prescriptions for metabolics (eg, lipid-lowering drugs) increased 109% among middle adults, and prescriptions for hematologics (eg, blood pressure drugs) increased 187% among the elderly [1].

Increased prescription drug costs have led to higher costs for both insurers and clients, resulting in more costly health insurance premiums for all consumers. Clients have responded to these increasing costs by not filling their prescriptions, taking less than the recommended dose, saving medications for future use, taking medicines belonging to other people, or using unprescribed alternative therapy. Any of these reactions may actually increase costs as a result of prolonged illness, loss of worker productivity, and hospitalization caused by inappropriate drug use, depending on the circumstances [8–10].

Consumers had more insurance coverage in 1999 than in 1985 and were more likely to purchase prescription drugs. In 1990, about 25% of prescriptions were paid for with private insurance. That number increased to 47% in 2001, with 31% of prescriptions paid for out-of-pocket, down from 59% in 1990. Medicaid paid 17% of prescription drug costs in 2001, whereas Medicare paid only 2%. This discrepancy is the basis for the current legislative debate over increasing Medicare prescription benefits coverage [1]. However, according to a landmark study in 2003, computerized retrospective-use review programs, used by all state Medicaid agencies and most private insurers for over a decade to prevent or rectify potential prescribing errors, have had no measurable effects on outpatient drug use or clinical outcomes in the Medicaid program. Policymakers must adopt a prospective approach (ie, reviewing prescriptions before a drug is dispensed) to seek ways to promote cost-effectiveness and minimize inappropriate prescribing for all forms of subsidies [11].

In the meantime, two states and several cities are starting to buy prescription drugs from Canada. Although new Medicare legislation signed by President Bush in December 2003 prohibits cross-border sales of drugs, citing legal and safety issues, these governors and mayors believe it would be unethical to wait, and expect to save their constituents as much as $1 million a year [12]. Recognizing the current economic pressures on all levels of government, particularly in the area of drug costs, an Institute of Medicine panel recently released a report that calls for universal health coverage by the year 2010, to align with the federal government's Healthy People 2010 initiative [13]. Before this issue is resolved, a future showdown is likely to occur among the players, including the US Department of Health and Human Services, the pharmaceutical industry, and state and city officials.

Because the elderly are more likely to have multiple ailments and require more prescriptions, there will be a significant continuing impact on prescription costs as the baby boom generation acquires Medicare coverage. In 1999, Medicare recipients' expenses were on average four times larger ($990) than non-Medicare beneficiaries ($236). The discrepancy between these mean drug expenses came primarily from differences in the quantities of drugs purchased rather than differences in prices paid for the drugs [14].

The 2001 National Ambulatory Medical Care Survey, a probability sample survey of visits to office-based health professionals in the United States, indicated that an average of 2.4 medications were ordered or provided at each office visit where particular drugs were mentioned. The leading therapeutic classes of drugs mentioned at office visits were cardiovascular-renal drugs and pain-relieving drugs. In office visits from 1992 through 2001, the leading diagnoses, therapeutic drug classes, and drug mentions drastically changed shape [15].

Variations in gender, age, ethnicity, and setting of prescription drug usage are significant. Research indicates relatively high rates of inappropriate prescription drug usage among white and African Americans aged 65 years and older, yet lower rates among Mexican Americans in the same age category [16]. Twenty percent of older, uninstitutionalized Americans are prescribed an inappropriate medication, often one of the 48 medicines that should never be prescribed for that age group [17,18]. With a few exceptions, the most significant predictors of inappropriate prescribing with regard to patients include polypharmacy, poor health status, and female sex [19]. Additionally, although surveys show that illicit drug use is primarily a problem among young males, excessive prescription drug use is predominantly a problem among middle-aged and older women in industrialized countries [20]. Findings also suggest that women, especially older women, may be prone to adverse effects as a result of unnecessarily high drug doses [21,22].

There has been a renewed interest in Therapeutic Drug Monitoring by health professionals worldwide as a result of the overall increase of prescription drugs, medication errors, and adverse drug reactions, and the call for quality-improvement evidence by state laws and accreditation agencies [23,24]. Recognition of pharmacodynamic variability and identification of pharmacokinetic parameters that best correlate with the clinical response have occurred in several areas including oncology, infection, and immunosuppression. In the future, genetic characteristics will be the basis of drug choice, dosage, and the likelihood of a response (pharmacogenetics) [25,26].

For now, trends in prescription drug use reflect a developing pattern of subtle, erratic disease and drug responses, influential consumer desires, variable prescribing practices, questionable drug promotion impacts, and diminishing drug purchase benefits, making the prescription drug arena a quagmire for even the quickest of decision-makers or the richest of consumers. For a closer look, this article groups representative types of prescription drug trends into four categories of drug use: health promotion, and primary, secondary, and tertiary prevention.

Health promotion drug use

Health promotion drugs are those prescribed to encourage or maintain a positive heath status, and include nutritional supplements such as vitamins, minerals, and herbs. Recent national surveys indicate that 70% of Americans take health promotion drugs because they feel the supplements provide them with energy and a feeling of wellness, or to help prevent illness or accelerate recovery when they are sick. More than 60% of people believe that food alone may not be enough to meet their nutritional goals. Those most likely to use daily supplements are women aged 60 to 74 years, while those least likely to be daily users are men aged 20 to 59 years [27,28].

Furthermore, older people who take supplements are more likely than nonusers to be physically active and to follow current dietary advice regarding salt, fat, cholesterol, sugar, caffeine, and fiber intake. If close to 50% of older adults receive dietary-supplement recommendations from their doctor, then prescribing supplement usage may be the way to promote positive attitudes about diet and health in older adults and others [27,28]. Because interactions have been confirmed between some prescribed drugs and supplements [29], health professionals need to incorporate supplement education and prescriptions into client care. Ironically, although supplement use is relatively high among health professionals, including doctors, nurses, dietitians, and pharmacists, it is often considered insignificant in the context of professional practice [28].

Primary prevention drug use

Primary prevention drugs are those prescribed to prevent problems or diseases. The most recognizable representatives of these drugs are vaccines. Sales of pediatric prophylactic vaccines are projected to increase from $3.3 billion to $5 billion by 2006, with sales of similar drugs for adults to increase from $2.3 billion to $3.8 billion. Therapeutic vaccines, possibly including one for AIDS, will likely garner only about 10% of the vaccine market [30].

Because half of all pneumonia-related deaths occur within the older population, the rates of influenza and pneumococcal disease vaccinations in this age group are revealing. Between 1989 and 1999, the number of noninstitutionalized older people who received a flu vaccination within the past year more than doubled, and between 1989 and 2001, the number of people within this same group who received pneumococcal vaccine increased from 14% to 54% [31]. But non-Hispanic whites are more likely to get flu vaccinations than are older African Americans and Hispanics, with an even greater disparity for pneumococcal vaccinations. The Centers for Disease Control and Prevention (CDC) reported that in 2001, flu shots were given to 65% of older non-Hispanic whites, 49% of African Americans, and 52% of Hispanics, and pneumococcal disease vaccinations were given to 58% of older non-Hispanic whites, 35% of African Americans, and 33% of Hispanics. This racial disparity motivated the Bush administration to launch a 2-year, $4 million outreach and vaccination program in four test cities and the Mississippi Delta. The recent increased demand for influenza vaccinations has only widened the disparity between the ethnic groups, because the rush for flu shots has mostly been within the suburban white population [32].

The controversy over mandatory pediatric vaccinations in our society continues, with a large antivaccination group arguing against the safety and efficacy of childhood vaccines. Several arguments are presented, including the assertions that: (1) vaccinations may weaken children's immune systems, (2) mercury-containing vaccines could cause neurological damage such as autism, (3) there is insufficient reporting of adverse reactions, (4) conflicts of interest exist where advisory committees have financial ties to the pharmaceutical companies that are producing the vaccines, (5) gate-keeping and tracking mechanisms are in place that remove parental choice, and (6) there is a lack of informed consent. A recent CDC report that, through the manipulation and stratification of data, made it seem as though the link between thimerosal (mercury)-containing vaccines and neurodevelopment disorders was eliminated, has further fueled mistrust and the sense of misinformation. Medical reviewers and a physician member of Congress have expressed concern regarding the tactics, ethics, and even the likelihood of conflicts of interest of the researchers [33–35].

The Vaccine Injury Compensation Program of 1986 insulates vaccine manufacturers from legal action, so safety–versus–profit is a significant consideration in a profit-driven health care system [35]. Whether this controversy will be resolved with public relations mechanisms, research-supported evidence, or both has yet to be determined. Meanwhile, vaccinations remain an integral part of disease-prevention measures, particularly in an era of bioterrorism and homeland security operations.

Other representative types of primary prevention drugs include lipid-lowering drugs and an antiplatelet drug (low-dose aspirin) that can prevent or substantially reduce the incidence of coronary heart disease and stroke in both young and old patients who remain on these medications for an average of 5 years. However, research shows that older patients tend to stop taking lipid-lowering statin drugs within 6 months after starting them and about 75% did not maintain drug therapy at a significant-enough level after 5 years. Among older patients, those less likely to continue long-term therapy were black, older than 75 years, had low income, had fewer cardiovascular problems when they began therapy, suffered from depression or dementia, or suffered from coronary heart disease problems such as heart attack after starting the therapy. Ironically, those who could benefit most from this type of prescribed therapy are often the ones who do not start or fail to continue the treatment [36]. As late as 2000, aspirin was prescribed to only 33% of clients who had coronary artery disease or a strong family history of heart disease or stroke [37]. A virtual rebellion is occurring in establishment medicine to translate research discoveries into life-saving and life-enhancing therapies, many of which involve prescription drugs.

Secondary prevention drug use

Secondary prevention drugs are related to early diagnosis and treatment. There are several representative types of secondary prevention drugs that have influenced prescription activity. Concern over microbial resistance to antibiotics, especially for *Streptococcus pneumoniae*, has increased over the last decade. In response, a new vaccine was developed to protect children from seven of the most invasive strains of *S pneumoniae* that cause more than 80% of serious infections.

Increased quantities of antibiotics prescribed to children for treatment of otitis media and upper respiratory infections (URIs) have contributed to antibiotic resistance. The CDC responded by actively promoting more judicious prescribing policies for children. As a result, antibiotic prescribing decreased as much as 12% between 1996 and 2000 [38–40]. Efforts from public health and professional organizations and the media to highlight and educate society about appropriate use of antibiotics contributed to this decrease. Paradoxically, with the decrease in antimicrobial prescribing for URIs in both children and adults, there was a proportional increase in prescribing broad-spectrum antibiotics for children [41]. Therefore, a shift, rather than a decrease, in antibiotic resistance may actually be occurring.

Another representative group of secondary prevention drugs showing a prescriptive change consists of cardiovascular drugs that are prescribed following acute myocardial infarction. The principles of evidence-based drug therapy for β-blockers, conclusively established in 1981 to save lives following heart attacks, are being applied in European and Scandinavian countries, but are lacking or delayed in the United States. β-Blockers were slow to be prescribed in the United States, with only 62.5% of eligible patients receiving prescriptions in 1996—15 years after proven evidence became available. Doctors are not totally at fault; among coronary artery disease patients questioned who were prescribed daily aspirin, only 60% took it in 1995, although this number increased to 80% by 1999 [37,42].

The misuse of drugs prescribed for legitimate purposes has been on the rise. This is particularly true for pain relievers, such as the opioid oxycodone group which is being diverted to the illicit drug market using fraudulent prescriptions, doctor-shopping, over-prescribing, and pharmacy theft [43,44]. This misuse had caused some health professionals to be cautious in prescribing analgesics, particularly controlled substances. Evidence also shows that health professionals and clients in the United States may have been indoctrinated to believe that certain pain medications are so dangerous and the need for control so essential, that client-access to appropriate pain relief is precarious. In the United Kingdom, the number of morphine prescriptions per capita is nearly twice that of the United States, and in Demark it is almost four times as high. Where addiction tends to occur, underuse of analgesics for acute pain is unrelated to recreational drug use for euphoria [45].

Other prescription drugs commonly associated with abuse are the benzodiazepines, in particular lorazepam (Ativan) and diazepam (Valium). Recent findings suggest that a significant number of women in substance-abuse rehabilitation programs may be dependent on anxiolytics in addition to other substances, requiring health professionals to scrutinize their use of these drugs in this treatment setting. This re-evaluation is especially necessary because there will be increased demand placed on the substance-abuse treatment programs in the future as a result of the number of aging baby boomers who have substance use and abuse problems [46,47].

The "war on drugs" has clearly failed, and in fact has resulted in some interesting paradoxes, such as an increase of HIV and tuberculosis infections in correctional institutions because of intravenous use, sexual practices, and close quarters with inadequate ventilation. Once individuals are released from incarceration, they are free to spread these diseases to their families and to the general public. Escalating federal expenditures to finance the war seem to have no clear end in sight [48–50]. If a change occurs in drug policy, such as controlled legalization and increased treatment for addiction, there will likely be an increase in prescriptive activity in this area, and the monies spent on the drug war could potentially be diverted to cover not only treatment programs but also legitimate prescription drug benefits.

Tertiary prevention drug use

Tertiary prevention drugs are designed to treat a disease state or injury and to prevent further progression. Chronic diseases have an annual economic cost to the United States of approximately $325 billion, a significant portion of it attributable to prescription drugs for conditions ranging from hay fever to heartburn and diabetes to depression [51].

Prescribing patterns of tertiary prevention drug use are important for a variety of reasons. Four chronic conditions—cardiovascular disease, cancer, chronic obstructive pulmonary disease, and diabetes—account for almost three quarters of all deaths in the United States. Medications for these conditions and other chronic diseases take a substantial amount of the research and development effort and will continue to direct the cost and number of available prescription drugs [52].

The market for new drugs in diabetic treatment, especially adult-onset diabetes, is fueled by statistics that indicate increasing rates of occurrence and longevity. Age-adjusted incidence of diagnosed diabetes in adults increased from 5.3% in 1997 to 6.5% in 2002. Adults aged 65 years and older are more than twice as likely to have diabetes as are adults aged 45 to 54 years. The number of visits to health practitioners' offices for individuals per population who had any diagnosis of diabetes ($N = 1000$) increased 35% for patients aged 45 to 54, and 43% for those aged 55 to 64 [53]. As of 2002, the total costs (both direct and indirect) of diabetes were estimated at $132 million. Among patients who had diabetes, 74.5% of those aged 18 to 44 years, 84.9% of those aged 45 to 64 years, 87.5% of those aged 65 to 74 years, and 86.6% of those aged 75 years and older were using some type of diabetic medication [54]. Along with traditional drugs (eg, insulin and oral antidiabetics), targeted drugs for insulin resistance (eg, metformin) are generating numerous prescriptions for diabetics and large profits for pharmaceutical companies [55].

In 2002, cancers cost this country over $170 billion, including more than $110 billion for lost productivity and over $60 billion for direct medical costs [56]. As the population ages and the number of people treated for cancer increases, prescription costs will likely increase proportionally. Medicare does not cover certain cancer care expenses, such as oral medicines commonly used to treat cancers of the breast and prostate. Out-of-pocket expenses add as much as 10% to the financial burden of cancer, and as new, more advanced, and more expensive treatments are adopted as standards of care, costs are estimated to increase exponentially [57]. Targeted drugs for cancer (eg, those that do not cure, but rather fight the disease without harming nearby healthy cells and therefore add years to life) have generated a phenomenally lucrative drug industry pipeline that will translate into a substantial prescription drug response and hefty costs. For example, there are more than 60 new cancer drugs available targeting angiogenesis that help decrease tumor growth by reducing the formation of new blood vessels [58,59].

Despite the existence of clinical guidelines to support appropriate use of prescription medications—particularly for asthma, congestive heart failure, and depression—underuse continues [60]. A recent study indicates that children who have prescriptions for one or more asthma drugs have fewer visits to the emergency room than those who have not been prescribed medications (most commonly African American and urban children who often have no prescription for a short-acting rescue drug to curb asthma attacks) [61].

A retrospective audit of patients who were diagnosed with congestive heart failure in a suburban community agency showed significant correlations between the number of medications prescribed, the number of inappropriate medications prescribed, the number of inappropriate dosages indicated, and the number of potential drug interactions. Multiple diagnoses did not make a difference [62]; about half of the patients suffering from depressive disorders, even HIV-positive medical patients, did not receive antidepressants, and psychotropic drug use was lower among African Americans than other ethnic groups [63].

Nonsteroidal anti-inflammatory drugs (NSAIDs), widely used to treat inflammation and pain in various conditions and frequencies, are pharmacologically diverse and include such agents as aspirin, ibuprofen, ketoprofen, and naproxen. Newer and costlier versions such as rofecoxib, meloxicam, and celecoxib are increasingly being prescribed, prompted by direct-to-consumer marketing. NSAIDs have varying side effects because they are chemically diverse, and yet they appear to have comparable efficacy. The greatest concern about NSAIDs relates to their gastrointestinal and renal effects, although reports also indicate adverse effects on mood, cognition, and behavior in patients who do not have psychiatric disorders. Children and older adults are particularly susceptible to hallucinosis, which occurs in a coherent state with awareness of having sensory misperceptions. This hallucinosis remits without residual side effects after discontinuation of the drug [64]. Regular use of over-the-counter NSAIDs is of concern because there is a lack of research regarding effectiveness. This research is usually conducted by drug companies, who have no financial incentive to test the long-term effectiveness of these drugs. Newer patented NSAIDs, on the other hand, are receiving rigorous testing, mostly to determine their benefit for specific diseases such as colon cancer and Alzheimer's disease [65].

Variable prescribing reflects a lack of consensus on NSAID use. There has been a reduction in prescribing NSAIDs for osteoarthritis because of increased risk for drug-induced complications and even death. The primary complication, gastrointestinal bleeding, is particularly common in older people. As a result of these indications, NSAID use decreased by 70%, and treatment costs were reduced by 53% over the last ten years [65]. General practitioners have challenged the latest study that indicates low-dose corticosteroids should be used instead of the costlier NSAIDs for rheumatoid arthritis. Meanwhile, very expensive new treatments, such as disease-modifying antirheumatic drugs are being developed [66].

Antihistamines, one of the most commonly used categories of medication and one of the fastest-growing sectors of the entire over-the-counter market [67], have a progressive history. First-generation antihistamines such as hydroxyzine are effective but cause sedation. Second-generation antihistamines such as loratadine and cetirizine have been effective in controlling allergic conditions without the sedation, although up to 23% of users may still feel sleepy when taking these drugs. More recently, third-generation antihistamines have been developed from existing agents (eg, desloratadine from loratadine and levocetirizine from cetirizine) to increase effectiveness and decrease side effects [68,69].

The recent release of some second-generation nonsedating antihistamines to over-the-counter status has prompted health insurers to end prescription drug coverage for clients or to raise the copay to the most expensive tier of coverage. Opponents of this move (eg, physician's groups such as the American College of Allergy, Asthma and Immunology, nonprofit research groups such as the Institute for Health and Productivity Management, and senior citizen groups such as the 60 Plus Association) have voiced strong concerns that reduced or eliminated coverage by managed care companies will result in most patients choosing to self-medicate using cheaper, over-the-counter first-generation sedating antihistamines, instead of more expensive second-generation ones that are better or more appropriate. Not only does this move undermine the client–provider partnership and create the possible misperception that health care providers are in agreement with this change, this action also causes safety and productivity concerns, particularly in the workplace where alertness and efficiency are crucial [70,71].

Strong arguments have been made that reducing or eliminating coverage of nonsedating antihistamines as a way to reduce the insurance companies' drug costs might actually cause an increase in overall management costs for patients' with chronic diseases. Recent research found that the newer drugs were associated with fewer hospitalizations and office visits and lower expenditures on nondrug care [70]. Addressing short-term gains rather than long-term benefits only adds to the overall costs of health care.

With herbal medicines becoming increasingly popular in the management of chronic disease, the likelihood of interaction between prescribed medications and herbal medicines is quite high. This interaction could either potentiate or antagonize the effects of the medications. Garlic, ginkgo biloba, ginseng, and St. John's wort have a significant influence on drugs taken concurrently, particularly drugs with narrow therapeutic windows. Older adults, the chronically ill, and the immunocompromised are particularly at risk for these interactions [72,73]. Future research will probably reveal more drug–herb relationships and provide better evidence-based decision-making.

Analysis of the Disability Follow-Back Survey, a supplement to the National Health Interview Surveys in 1994 and 1995, found that 1.3 million adults with disabilities reported health problems caused by not taking their medications as prescribed because of the high cost. Noncompliance in taking drugs occurred as a result of severe disability, poor health, low income, lack of insurance, and a high number of prescriptions. Yet most of the present proposals for expanding Medicare coverage do not offer special provisions to help the chronically ill or disabled [9].

Many citizen groups and health care professionals advocate for restructuring the health care delivery system from one with an acute-care focus to one with a chronic-care focus, and suggest that the education of health professionals, the way in which care is provided, and how health services are paid for should be re-evaluated [74]. Whether that paradigm shift occurs or not, the trend toward chronic care is inevitable from the prescription drug perspective, at least until the baby boom generation passes into history. How we take care of the younger generations and how they take care of themselves are likely to determine whether that paradigm change will be temporary or permanent.

Discussion

Clearly, there is an overall increase in prescription drug use for a multitude of reasons, even though there are specific categories of drugs with decreased or episodic variance (Table 1). There is a need for targeted and timely health information, including medication management, so that clients can achieve their desired therapeutic results. This approach is called "information therapy" or providing "information prescriptions" [75]. A recent survey revealed that more than 75% of clients and health professionals believe the inability to understand information about prescription medications, a form of low health-literacy, contributes to poor health outcomes. Reasons for low health-literacy include difficulty reading, language barriers, a feeling of intimidation or vulnerability, and reluctance to admit a lack of understanding [76]. A study from Denmark showed that clients may be confused by inconsistent information provided in leaflets about different brands of generic drugs [77]. This may likely be the case for the United States market as well, as most pharmaceutical corporations are international in scope.

Some suggested remedies for low health-literacy include [76,78,79]:

- Teaching information about the pharmaceutical industry to students in health professions, as attitudes are formed before graduation;
- Coordinating drug makers' information to reduce client confusion;
- Improving information access for health care institutions and pharmacies;

- Making communication with clients a priority for all health professionals;
- Encouraging legible prescriptions (mandated by law in two states so far).

The Agency for Healthcare Research and Quality and the National Council on Patient Information and Education have responded to this concern by developing a fill-in guide for clients to promote safe medication administration [80].

In 2001 the Institute of Medicine (IOM) released a report entitled "Crossing the Quality Chasm: A New Health System for the 21st Century" in which the panel stated:

> The current system often requires a visit as the only legitimate format of care and, more important, as the only form of professional work that is compensated and measured in the health care world as 'productivity.' The product of health care is not visits or 'encounters' but healing relationships that allow patients to obtain the trustworthy information and support they need [81].

Table 1
Trends based on representative types of drugs showing prescriptive change

Category	Decreasing	Variable	Increasing
Health promotion			
Nutritional supplements		X	
Primary prevention			
Prophylactic vaccines		X	
Lipid-lowering drugs		X	
Antiplatelet (aspirin)		X	
Secondary prevention			
Antimicrobials	X		
Broad-spectrum antibiotics			X
Beta-blockers		X	
Opioids		X	
Anxiolytics		X	
Tertiary prevention			
Insulin and oral antidiabetics			X
Targeted diabetic drugs			X
Oral breast and prostate cancer drugs		X	
Targeted cancer drugs			X
Asthma drugs		X	
Congestive heart failure drugs		X	
Antidepressants		X	
NSAIDs (includes aspirin)		X	
Antihistamines			
First generation	X		
Second generation			X
Third generation			X
Herbals			X

Achieving healing relationships requires shared decision-making, defined as "a process in which both the patient and the clinician/team share information with each other, take steps to participate in the decision-making process, and agree on a course of action." [82] Shared decision-making promotes client autonomy; trust; and knowledge about options, benefits and harms; and reduces decisional conflict. Because of insufficient research and the fact that all parties must agree to be involved, it is not yet known whether shared decision-making improves health outcomes [82].

Nurses have long known the benefit of shared decision-making and have much to communicate to other health professionals. But considering the climate of the unrelenting nursing shortage, nurses have less time, energy, and motivation to devote to educating other health professionals. Yet the time has come for all health professionals to practice this concept.

According to the IOM panel, barriers to clients' participation in shared decision- making include confusion between problem solving and decision-making, realization that health care is an inexact science, not understanding the need to make a decision, resistance to a new role in one's own care, no appreciation of client autonomy because of ethnic membership, and regret of decisions with bad outcomes. The IOM panel also indicated that barriers to health professionals using shared decision-making include competition for shared decision-making time, absence of financial reimbursements, lack of training in shared decision-making techniques, and the need for system-level changes in how health professionals engage clients [82].

A challenge for both clients and health providers is the need for medical interpretation, which reduces error by improving communication. In 2002, an Access Project study reported that 27% of clients who had no interpreter left the hospital not knowing how to take their medication, compared with 2% of those who had an interpreter [83]. By law, any agency receiving federal funding is required to provide interpreting services. Medical interpretation issues are slowly being remedied in community settings (only one in five clinics currently do not offer any type of interpreting services), but hospital settings are still limping along because of cost containment mandates [84,85]. As our country becomes more culturally diverse, drug prescribing will become increasingly challenging.

Summary

Prescribing practices are a reflection of health professionals' abilities to discriminate among the various choices of drugs and determine the ones that will most benefit their patients. As selective as practitioners must be, they cannot limit themselves to knowing only those drugs that fit within the dominant paradigm of acute care. They must broaden their exposure to incorporate knowledge of drugs that permeate clients' lives through media and self-administration. Health promotion drug use is just emerging as a prescriptive activity, but it will become more significant in the future. Primary and secondary prevention drug uses are in flux, and tertiary prevention drug use is likely to overwhelm our system, particularly with the baby boom generation, until our society can switch its focus to more health promotion and disease prevention. It is imperative that health professionals develop shared decision-making capabilities for client education and appropriate prescribing. Only when the health care system exhibits a true client–provider partnership will the "five rights"—right drug, right dose, right route, right time, right client—be accurately applied. With the increasing and overwhelming costs of prescription drugs, health practitioners cannot afford to sit idle; as professionals and stakeholders, they must engage health policy makers and persuade these entities to share their concerns and views, and help their clients, the profession, and themselves.

References

[1] Centers for Disease Control and Prevention. National Health Care Survey News Clippings page. Available at: http://www.cdc.gov/about/major/nhcs/nhcs_newsclippings.html. Accessed November 4, 2003.

[2] Siegel M. Fighting the drug ad wars: as corporations push new medicines, sound and affordable healthcare suffers. Nation 2002;274(23):21.

[3] Curious and confused: prescription drug ads impact consumer health [editorial]. Medical Letter on the CDC & FDA. Fayetteville: University of Arkansas; November 2, 2003.

[4] Kaiser Family Foundation. Understanding the effects of direct-to-consumer prescription drug advertising. Available at: http://www.kff.org/content/2001/3197/DTC%20Ad%20 Survey.pdf. Accessed December 12, 2004.

[5] Rosenthal MB, Berndt ER, Donohue JM, et al. Demand effects of recent changes in prescription drug promotion. Available at: http://www.kff.org. Accessed December 12, 2004.

[6] President Bush signs reauthorization of PDUFA [news briefs]. Drug Utilization Review Newsletter 2002;18(8):62.

[7] New CDC study claims sharp increases in prescription rates across all ages & in nearly all specialties: at current rate, drug spending would double in next 5 years. Biomedical Market Newsletter 2002;12(5):21.

[8] Mitchell J, Mathews HF, Hunt LM, et al. Mismanaging prescription medications among rural elders: the effects of socioeconomic status, health status, and medication profile indicators. Gerontologist 2001;41(3):348–56.

[9] Kennedy J, Erb C. Prescription noncompliance due to cost among adults with disabilities in the United States. Am J Public Health 2002;92(7):1120–4.

[10] Higher out-of-pocket costs cause massive noncompliance in the use of prescription drugs, and this is likely to grow. Medical Benefits 2003;20(4):5.

[11] Hennessy S, Strom BL. The ineffectiveness of retrospective drug utilization review. LDI Issue Brief 2003;9(1):1–4.

[12] First state is set to buy Canadian drugs. Pharma Marketletter. Dec 15, 2003.

[13] Committee on the Consequences of Uninsurance. Insuring America's health: principles and recommendations, The National Academies Press. Available at: http://www.nap.edu. Accessed January 21, 2004.

[14] Chartbook #12: outpatient prescription drug expenses of 1999. Agency for Healthcare Research and Quality. December 2003. Available at: http://www.meps.ahrq.gov/papers/ cb12.htm. Accessed January 20, 2004.

[15] Cherry DK, Burt CW, Woodwell DA. National ambulatory medical care survey: 2001 summary. Adv Data 2003;337:1–44.

[16] Raji MA, Ostir GV, Markides KS, et al. Potentially inappropriate medication use by elderly Mexican Americans. Ann Pharmacother 2003;37(9):1197–202.

[17] Agency for Healthcare Research and Quality. AHRQ focus on research: pharmaceutical research highlights, Available at: http://www.ahrq.gov/news/focus/phrmhigh.htm. Accessed January 19, 2004.

[18] Beers criteria for medications to avoid in the elderly are updated. Health & Med Week. Dec 29, 2003:262.

[19] Liu GG, Christensen DB. The continuing challenge of inappropriate prescribing in the elderly: an update of the evidence. J Am Pharm Assoc (Wash) 2002;42(6):847–57.

[20] Adrian M. How can sociological theory help our understanding of addictions? Subst Use Misuse 2003;38(10):1385–423.

[21] Cohen JS. Do standard doses of frequently prescribed drugs cause preventable adverse effects in women? J Am Med Womens Assoc 2002;57(2):105–10, 113.

[22] Lewis G. Polypharmacy and older people. Nurs Times 2003;99(17):54–5.

[23] Schulz M, Schmoldt A. Therapeutic and toxic blood concentrations of more than 800 drugs and other xenobiotics. Pharmazie 2003;58(7):447–74.

[24] Benjamin DM, Pendrak RF. Medication errors: an analysis comparing PHICO's closed claims data and PHICO's event reporting trending system (PERTS). J Clin Pharmacol 2003; 43(7):754–9.

[25] Thomson AH. Individualization of drug dosage – past, present and future. Med Monatsschr Pharm 2003;26(5):150–2.

[26] Nicol MJ. The variation of response to pharmacotherapy: pharmacogenetics – a new perspective to 'the right drug for the right person.' Medsurg Nurs 2003;12(4):242–9.

[27] Fazio M. Equipment 101: a tableting perspective: an overview of the opportunities and challenges in the dietary supplement market. Nutraceuticals World 2003;6(19):S13–4.

[28] Informed consumers recognize supplements' benefits. MMR 2003;20(6):24–5.

[29] President and Fellows of Harvard College. Herbs and dietary supplements. Alternative Medicine (Harvard Special Health Reports), 2001. Available at: http://galenet.galegroup. com/servlet/HWRC/htm. Accessed January 19, 2004.

[30] Black H. Vaccine vitality generates jobs. Scientist 2001;15(18):35.

[31] Zimmerman RK, Mieczkoedki TA, Wilson SA. Immunization rates and beliefs among elderly patients of inner city neighborhood health centers. Health Promo Prac 2002;3(2): 197–206.

[32] Borenstein S. CDC aims to end racial disparities in adult vaccinations. Knight Ridder/ Tribune News Service. Dec 11, 2003:K2503.

[33] Sheppard J. Vaccinations: a parent's right to choose. Available at: http://healthychild.com/ database/vaccinations_a_parent_s_right_to_choose.htm. Accessed November 24, 2003.

[34] Fazackerley A. When fear becomes another epidemic. Times Higher Ed Supp 2003;0(1619): 20.

[35] O Meara KP. CDC study raises level of suspicion. Insight on the News. Feb 3, 2004.

[36] Benner JS, Glynn RJ, Mogun MS, et al. Long-term persistence in use of statin therapy in elderly patients. JAMA 2002;288(4):455–61.

[37] Lenfant C. Shattuck lecture: clinical research to clinical practice – lost in translation? N Engl J Med 2003;349(9):868–74.

[38] New community-based study tracks rates of antibiotic-resistant bacteria in Massachusetts children [press release]. Rockville: Agency for Healthcare Research and Quality; October 6, 2003. Available at: http://www.ahrq.gov/news/press/pr2003/mabactpr.htm. Accessed October 20, 2003.

[39] Centers for Disease Control and Prevention. Diagnosis and management of acute pharyngitis in children. Continuing Education Course, September 26, 2003. Available at: http://www.cdc.gov/drugresistance/community/htm. Accessed October 20, 2003.

[40] Finkelstein JA, Stille D, Nordin J, et al. Reduction in antibiotic use among US children, 1996–2000. Pediatrics 2003;112(3 Pt 1):620–7.

[41] Mainous AG 3rd, Hueston WJ, Davis MP, et al. Trends in antimicrobial prescribing for bronchitis and upper respiratory infections among adults and children. Am J Public Health 2003;93(11):1910–4.

[42] Reikvam A, Kvan E, Aursnes I. Use of cardiovascular drugs after acute myocardial infarction: a marked shift towards evidence-based drug therapy. Cardiovasc Drugs Ther 2002;16(5):451–6.

[43] Meadows M. Prescription drug use and abuse. FDA Consum 2001;35(5):18–24.

[44] Dumas LG, Hennessey Wohn MB. Substance abuse. In: Hitchcock JE, Schubert PE, Thomas SA, editors. Community health nursing: caring in action. 2nd edition. Clifton Park, NY: Delmar Learning; 2003. p. 817–52.

[45] Herrera S. The morphine myth. Forbes 1997;159(10):258–60.

[46] Cormier RA. The use of tranquillizers among women undergoing substance abuse treatment. Can J Nurs Res 2003;35(1):74–82.

[47] Gfroerer J, Penne M, Pemberton M, et al. Substance abuse treatment need among older adults in 2020: the impact of the aging baby-boom cohort. Drug Alcohol Depend 2003;69(2): 127–35.

[48] Clark CF, Knox MD. Effective drug enforcement and HIV transmission: a modern paradox. AIDS Patient Care 1991;5(4):168–72.

[49] Skolnick AA. Some experts suggest the nation's 'War on Drugs' is helping tuberculosis stage a deadly comeback. JAMA 1992;268(22):3177–9.

[50] Massing M. Home-court advantage: what the war on drugs teaches us about the war on terrorism. Am Prospect 2001;12(21):24–8.

[51] Centers for Disease Control and Prevention. Chronic Disease Overview. Available at: http://www.cdc.gov/nccdphp/overview.htm. Accessed January 30, 2004.

[52] Health care in the 21st century: slow focus shift to chronic ills [editorial]. Med Health 2001; 55(36):7.

[53] Centers for Disease Control and Prevention. Diabetes Public Health Resource. Percent of adults with diabetes using diabetes medication, by age, United States, 1997–2002. Available at: http://www.cdc.gov/nccdphp/diabetes/index.htm. Accessed January 16, 2004.

[54] Centers for Disease Control and Prevention. Highlights from trend tables and chartbook. Available at: http://www.cdc.gov/nchs/hus.htm. Accessed October 20, 2003.

[55] Companies brace for diabetes market battle after drug review [editorial]. Med Mark Media 1999;34(6):22.

[56] Centers for Disease Control and Prevention. Preventing chronic diseases: investing wisely in health. Screening to prevent cancer deaths. Available at: http://www.cdc.gov/nccdphp.htm. Accessed January 21, 2004.

[57] National Cancer Institute. 2001 Cancer Progress Report. Costs of Cancer Care. Available at: http://progressreport.cancer.gov/doc.htm. Accessed January 21, 2004.

[58] Lau G. Competition heats up for new cancer drugs. Investor's Business Daily. July 1, 2003:A06.

[59] Hampton T. Cancer researchers target angiogenesis. JAMA 2003;290(19):2529–32.

[60] Gilberg K, Laouri M, Wade S, et al. Analysis of medication use patterns: apparent overuse of antibiotics and under-use of prescription drugs for asthma, depression, and CHF. J Manag Care Pharm 2003;9(3):232–7.

[61] University of Michigan Health System. Study: kids who get prescription asthma drugs visit ER less often; but black, urban kids make more frequent emergency visits. Ascribe Higher Education News Service. May 6, 2003.

[62] Gallagher LP. Research brief: the potential for adverse drug reactions in elderly patients. Appl Nurs Res 2001;14(4):220–4.

[63] Vitiello B, Burnam MA, Bing EG, et al. Use of psychotropic medications among HIV-infected patients in the United States. Am J Psychiatry 2003;160(3):547–54.

[64] Sussman N. Psychiatric manifestations of NSAIDS in older adults. Psychiatric Times December 1, 2002;26.

[65] Stipp D. Scientists believe they may have found a common link in diseases from cancer to Alzheimer's to heart disease. Here's the story behind the search for THE SECRET KILLER. Fortune 2003;148(19):108.

[66] GPs challenge latest study on use of corticosteroids. GP. February 3, 2003:20.

[67] Feverish activity. Chemist & Druggist. May 25, 2002:18.

[68] Scheinfeld N. The new antihistamines – desloratadine and levocetirizine: a review. J Drugs Dermatol 2002;1(3):311–7.

[69] Antihistamines reviewed. Chemist & Druggist. August 24, 2002:21.

[70] Experts concerned about insurance coverage of second generation antihistamines. Health & Med Week. October 6, 2003;34.

[71] Levy S. IHPM to health plans: don't end coverage for allergy meds. Drug Topics 2002; 146(21):52.

[72] Clinicians must remain alert for interactions between herbal medicines and prescribed drugs [editorial]. Drugs Ther Perspect 2002;18(9):17–21.

[73] Awang DVC, Fugh-Berman A. Herbal interactions with cardiovascular drugs. J Cardiovasc Nurs 2002;16(4):64–70.

[74] Health care in the 21st century: slow focus shift to chronic ills [editorial]. Med Health 2001; 55(36):7.

[75] Mettler M, Kemper DW. Information therapy: health education one person at a time. Health Promot Pract 2003;4(3):214–7.

[76] Study: failure to understand prescription drug information contributes to poor health outcomes [editorial]. Health Care Strateg Manage 2002;20(11):8–9.

[77] Bjerrum L, Foged A. Patient information leaflets – helpful guidance or a source of confusion? Pharmacoepidemiol Drug Saf 2003;12(1):55–9.

[78] Monaghan MS, Galt KA, Turner PD, et al. Student understanding of the relationship between the health professions and the pharmaceutical industry. Teach Learn Med 2003; 15(1):14–20.

[79] Florida mandates legible Rxs. Drug Topics 2003;147(15):5.

[80] Agency for Healthcare Research and Quality and National Council on Patient Information and Education. Your medicine: play it safe. Available at: http://www.ahrq.gov/consumer/safemeds/safemeds.htm. Accessed May 6, 2003.

[81] Institute of Medicine of the National Academies. Crossing the quality chasm: a new health system for the 21st century. Available at: http://www.iom.edu/report.htm. Accessed January 16, 2004.

[82] Sheridan SL, Harris RP, Woolf SH. Shared decision-making about screening and chemoprevention: a suggested approach from the US Preventive Services Task Force. Am J Prev Med 2004;26(1):56–66.

[83] Access Project. What a difference an interpreter can make: health care experiences of uninsured with limited English proficiency. Available at: http://www.accessproject.org/camspublications.htm. Accessed January 25, 2004.

[84] Kaneya R. Hospitals, clinics lack interpreters. The Chicago Reporter 2002;31(8):3–7.

[85] Bartoo CH. Study shows electronic prescriptions safer for kids. Vanderbilt University Medical Center Reporter, January 9, 2004:1,4.

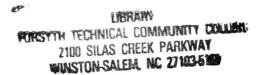

ELSEVIER
SAUNDERS

Nurs Clin N Am 40 (2005) 51–62

NURSING
CLINICS
OF NORTH AMERICA

Strategies for Acquiring Affordable Medications for Seniors

Kathy J. Morris, RN, MSN, ARNP, FNP-BC

*Council Bluffs Community Health Center, 300 West Broadway,
Suite 6, Council Bluffs, IA, 51503, USA*

The story is not a new one; it appears on television and in newspapers, and the issue is repeatedly debated in state and national legislatures. The names and locations change, but the message remains the same: senior citizens cannot afford their medications [1–3]. Many seniors have even returned to work in effort to pay their monthly prescription bills. Many senior citizens find themselves having to choose which medications they can afford to take, and others are unable to pay for both medication and food [4].

People are now living longer. The 2000 census recorded 35 million people over the age of 65, representing a 12% increase since 1990, and the census bureau predicts this growth will continue [5]. The increasing population of seniors is draining an already strained Medicare system. Health declines with advancing age, and pharmaceutic care becomes an important part of seniors' health care management. Many seniors who cannot afford their medications simply do not take them. This causes complications for patients with chronic health problems, and these complications then increase emergency department and hospital visits, which in turn increases the Medicare burden. When evaluating long-term health costs of the senior population, it is important to consider that if compliance with medication regimes promotes improved health in this group, making medications affordable can prove to be cost-effective for the health care system [6].

Many patients over the age of 65 require three to five medications per day. This is a conservative estimate, as it is not unusual for some seniors with multiple chronic illnesses to take ten or more daily medications. The total annual medication bill for United States senior citizens averages $3 billion [7], and the cost of prescription drugs continues to increase, further compounding the problem. Between 1993 and1998, the cost of drugs increased an was average of 40%, and this inflation is predicted to continue on an upward curve with no end in sight [4]. Although some individuals

0029-6465/05/$ - see front matter © 2005 Elsevier Inc. All rights reserved.
doi:10.1016/j.cnur.2004.09.013
nursing.theclinics.com

have prescription coverage, approximately 35% of senior citizens do not [8]. Even seniors with prescription coverage see increases in their copayments as insurance providers scramble to maintain benefits [9].

Data from the Health and Retirement Study indicates that over a 2-year period, 2 million Medicare beneficiaries were noncompliant with medication regimens as a result of drug costs [11]. Some undermedicated by skipping doses or pill cutting, whereas others simply did not fill prescriptions [6,7]. Medication noncompliance, especially in patients who have hypertension, diabetes, and heart disease, has been linked to an increase in complications, emergency department visits, and hospital admissions. Seniors who have multiple medical problems and cannot afford their complete medication regimen must choose which medication is the most important for them to take, often without understanding the implications of their decision. The demographic and socio-economic factors related to medication noncompliance that have been studied include: age, sex, extent of insurance coverage, and out-of-pocket costs [2]. All of these issues are relevant to the senior population. The majority of seniors are women who have greater financial burdens than men. Although many of these women had been in the workforce, women's employer-based retirement plans were less likely to have drug benefits than men's [12]. The ongoing noncompliance problem has societal implications: the resulting increase in emergency department visits and hospitalizations can eventually lead to more nursing home placements and consequently increase Medicare and Medicaid costs [13]. Another important consideration is the decreased quality of life for noncompliant seniors.

Some resources and options are available to help make the older patient's monthly medication bill a little more affordable, but many seniors are unaware of or unable to locate these resources. Some senior citizens are afraid to tell their physicians [6] and children [10] that they cannot afford their medication, and therefore they either skip their medications or incur a significant credit card debt. This article addresses the problem and identifies the resources available to nurses and patients.

Legislative action

After years of work in the legislature, President Bush recently signed new Medicare legislation that addresses prescription drugs issues. The Medicare Prescription Drug, Improvement, and Modernization Act was signed into law in 2003. Although the new prescription benefit will not be completely in effect until 2006, seniors may obtain a discount drug card during the interim. This card is intended to reduce the retail costs of medications from 10% to 25% [14,15]. Additionally, seniors with lower income (ie, $12,124 for singles and $16,363 for married couples in 2004) will qualify for an additional $600 credit on their prescription card [16]. By paying a premium of approximately

$35, Medicare beneficiaries may opt to enroll in a plan that covers prescription drugs. The plans offered may differ, but all have common characteristics. For example, current plans call for the beneficiary to pay the first $250 of prescription drugs cost, which is considered a deductible. Medicare will then pay 75% of drugs costs between $250 and $2,250, while the senior pays the other 25%. When the $2,250 limit is reached, the senior pays 100% of the drug costs until the $3,600 out-of-pocket spending limit is reached. After that $3,600 limit is reached, Medicare will pay 95% of prescription drug costs. Different plans may include further options to help pay the out-of-pocket expenses [17].

The dilemma facing senior citizens has not gone unnoticed at the state level. Maine recently initiated a prescription card program for its citizens. The program is not limited to seniors, but is based on income. Enrollment began in summer 2004, with eligibility based on the federal poverty levels. Maine is not the only state addressing the problem. Twenty-five states have some type of plan in place for prescription drug assistance (Table 1) [18–21]. The American Association of Retired Persons (AARP) also provides a list of state-sponsored prescription drug discount programs on their Web site [22].

Legislators in some of the northern Midwestern states, including Illinois, Maine, and Minnesota, are endorsing legalization that would permit importation of lower-cost medications from Canada, claiming that the lower-cost drugs could then be used for a state-supported drug program for seniors. Some states attempt to assist seniors by providing Web sites where prescription medications can be ordered from Canada, or even sponsor bus trips to Canada to enable seniors to make over-the-border medication purchases [23].

The FDA and several pharmaceutical companies are working to stop the importation of prescription medications. The FDA is taking action against companies that help seniors buy Canadian drugs over the internet, United States Customs agencies are confiscating imported medications, and pharmaceutical companies are threatening to stop shipments to Canadian pharmacies unless sales to United States seniors are discontinued. Although a bipartisan bill was introduced in the Senate to prevent drug companies from cutting off supplies to Canadian pharmacies that sell to American seniors [24], it was still illegal to import drugs from other countries as of fall 2004 [18,20,21].

Generic medications

One of the most common methods of controlling medication costs is the use of generic medications. As drug costs continue to climb, private insurance companies and Medicaid drug programs have been evaluating the use of generic medications. In 2000, a study evaluating the use of generics in

Table 1
State sponsored prescription drug discount programs

State	Qualifications	Income restrictions	Plan	Cost to join	Information
California	Medicare beneficiaries	None	Discounts the same as Med-Cal	None	HICAP 800-434-0222
Connecticut	Low income >65 or disabled	Yes	Most drugs 30-d supply for $12	$25/y	Department of Social Services 800-423-5026
Delaware	>65 or disabled	Yes	State pays 75% of drug costs to $2500/y with $5 copay	None	Division of Social Services 800-996-9969
Florida Prescription Assistance Program for Seniors	>65 who are eligible for Medicare Savings Program	Yes	$80/mo of prescription drugs with $10 copay	None	Agency for Health Care Administration 800-963-5337
Florida Medicare Prescription Discount Program	Medicare beneficiaries	None	Medicare card receives discount	None	Agency for Health Care Administration 800-963-5337
Illinois	>65 or disabled	Yes	Restricted by income and medications for specific diseases with variable copay	$5–$25	Department of Revenue 800-624-2459
Indiana	>65 without drug coverage	Yes	Refunds on prescriptions between $500–$1000 annually	None	HoosieRX 866-267-4679
Iowa	Medicare beneficiaries	None	Discount card varying discounts on certain drugs	$20/y	Iowa Priority Prescription Savings Program 866-282-5817

State	Eligibility		Benefits	Fee	Contact
Kansas	>67 eligible for Medicare and without drug coverage	Yes	Reimbursement for 70% out-of-pocket cost, $1200/y cap	None	Department of Aging 785-368-7327
Maryland	>65	Yes	Discount card With copay	$10/mo	CareFirst 800-972-4612
Massachusetts	>65 and some disabled	Yes	Deductible $2000–$3000, then 100% covered	None	Office of Elder Affairs 800-243-4636
Michigan	Low income >65	Yes	Most prescriptions covered, copay varies by income	$25 application fee	Currently closed except emergency coverage 866-747-8444
Minnesota	>65 enrolled in state Medicare supplement	Yes	$35/mo out-of-pocket, then covered 100%	None	Senior LinkAge Line 800-333-2433
Nevada	>62	Yes	Copay with state paying up to $5000/y	None	Senior Rx 800-262-7726
New Hampshire	>65	None	Discount card 15% off brand-name, 40% generic	None	New Hampshire Prescription Drug Discount 888-580-8902
New Jersey The Pharmaceutical Assistance to the Aged and Disabled	>65 or disabled	Yes	Discount card with $5 copay at participating pharmacies	None	Department of Health and Human Services 800-792-9745
New Jersey Senior Gold Prescription Discount	>65 disabled	Yes	Discount card with $15 copay	None	Department of Health and Human Services
North Carolina	>65	Yes	Discount card with maximum	None	Department of Health and Human Services 800-662-7030
Pennsylvania PACENET	>65	Yes	$500 deductible and copay	None	Pennsylvania Department of Aging 800-225-7223

(continued on next page)

Table 1 *(continued)*

State	Qualifications	Income restrictions	Plan	Cost to join	Information
Rhode Island RIPAE	Low/moderate income >65	Yes	Discount card saves 15%–60%	None	Department of Elder Affairs 401-222-2880
South Carolina	Low income >65	Yes	$500 deductible and copay	None	SILVERx CARE 877-239-5277
Vermont VHAP	Low income >65	Yes	Discount card and copay	None	Vermont Health Access 800-529-4060
Vermont VSCRIPT	>65 or disabled	Yes	Medications for long-term medical problems	None	Vermont Health Access 800-529-4060
Vermont VSCRIPT Expanded	Moderate income >65	Yes	Discount card Copay 41% per script	None	Vermont Health Access 800-529-4060
Wyoming	All state residents	Yes	Copay limited to 3 drugs/mo	None	Division of Family Services 800-442-2766

Data from Refs. [30–33].

49 states identified a potential savings of $229 million over a 1-year period [25]. Many insurance companies now offer tiered copays, with a lower copay offered to customers who use generic drugs [26]. The number of available generic medications is rapidly increasing as many brand-name drugs have reached the end of their patents. Patent expirations were expected on more than 100 brand-name drugs in 2003 [27].

Generic drugs have been mistrusted in the past, but it is important to note that the FDA approves the bioequivalence of generic drugs. All but a few generics provide therapeutic benefits identical to their brand-name counterparts. In an attempt to promote patient confidence in generics, the FDA supported a consumer information campaign in 2003, posting public service advertisements on buses and in consumer magazines [28].

Major pharmaceutical companies have encouraged the distrust of generics by misinforming physicians about the quality of these drugs. Combined with the free samples generously given to health care providers, this has promoted the use of brand-name drugs. A common practice by pharmaceutical companies is to introduce a new formulation or an improved version of the brand-name drug when the patent expires, which encourages continued use of the brand-name drug. The cost of brand-name drugs can be as high as four times the cost of the generic versions, but this depends on the available competition; if only one company is making a generic drug, the cost of the two versions may not be much different [28,29].

Resources

Pharmaceutical companies are not insensitive to the needs of senior citizens. Many companies have discount cards that can be used at local pharmacies [30–33]. Some programs offer a Web site where medications can be ordered, and others allow medications to be mail-ordered. All of the programs have income requirements for eligibility, most of which are based on the poverty level (Table 2) [32,33]. Another option offered by some companies is the Medical Assistance Programs (MAP), where eligible patients submit the required paper work and prescriptions from their health care provider and receive a 3-month supply of their medication for a discounted price. The MAP programs are not widely advertised and are usually only available through direct contact with the pharmaceutical company [32]. It is important for patients to understand that they need to discuss these programs with their health care provider, and request written prescriptions and assistance with applications to take advantage of the benefits. Patients may also request to have their medication changed to a brand that offers an assistance program. Financial status needs to be discussed with health care providers so that medication costs can be considered when choosing regimens. Box 1 lists some internet sites that help in finding patient assistance programs.

Table 2
Pharmaceutical company drug discount cards

Company	Name of program	Income restrictions	Plan	Contact information
Eli Lilly	LillyAnswers Card	$18,000/Individual $24,000/Household	$12 per prescription at participating pharmacies	877-795-4559 www.lillyanswers.com
GlaxoSmithKline	Orange Card	$26,000/Individual $35,000/Couple	30%–40%savings on drugs at participating pharmacies	888-672-6436 www.gsk.com
Novaritis	Together Rx	Two levels: 1) $18,000/Individual $24,000/Couple 2) $24,000/Individual $38,000/Couple	Two level: 1) $12/mo per prescription 2) 25%–40% discounts both options must be used at participating pharmacies	866-974-2273 www.NovartisCarePlan.com
Pfizer New Program	Connection to Card	$19,000/Individual $31,000/Couple	Eligible patients my receive free medicines at some physicians offices	888-717-6005 www.pfizerforliving.com
Pfizer New Program	Pfriends	$31,000/Individual $45,000/Couple	Families below the income level receive 37%–50% off average cash price; Families above the income level may receive 15%–25% off average cash price	800-717-6005 www.pfizerforliving.com
Pfizer	Share Card	$18,000/Individual $24,000/Couple	$15/mo per prescription at participating pharmacies	800-717-6005 www.pfizerforliving.com
Multiple companies: Abbott, AstraZeneca Aventis, Bristol-Meyers Squibb, GlaxoSmithKline, Johnson & Johnson, Novartis	Together Rx Card	$28,000/Individual $38,000/Couple	20%–40% discounts at participating pharmacies for various medications	800-865-7211 www.together-rx.com

Data from Refs. [30–33].

Box 1. Internet resources for patient assistance programs

http://www.canadapharmacy.com: Canadian mail order pharmacy

http://www.needymeds.com: Free resource that searches pharmaceutical companies for drugs needed

http://www.rxassist.org: A site for health care providers supported through Robert Wood Johnson Foundation

http://www.medicare.gov/Prescription/Home.asp: Medicare website that identifies drug assistance programs and state- and community-based programs

http://www.va.gov/vbs/health or http://www.tricare.osd.mil/ retirees: Site for veterans, military retired, and widowed spouses

http://www.freemedicineprogram.com: Helps consumers enroll in medication assistance programs

http://www.BenefitsCheckUp.org: National Council of Aging site listing state-funded pharmacies and company-sponsored assistance programs

http://www.ncsl.org/programs/health/drugs340b.htm: Community Health Centers and other organizations that have access to low cost medications

---

AARP is also an important resource and advocate for senior citizens. The AARP Web sites provide updates on current legislation, and tips for health, finance, and travel. Seniors struggling with prescription costs should be encouraged to make contact with AARP [34,35].

Splitting pills

Splitting or cutting pills can also be an effective cost-savings method. Many pharmaceutical companies have level pricing, which means that even when the strength of the medication increases, the cost does not. Therefore, sometimes 2-months' worth of mediation can be purchased for the price of a 1-month quantity by obtaining the higher strength of the medication and cutting the pills into lower-strength portions. Studies have shown that patients can save between $600 and $700 per year on specific medications using this method. Some medications conducive to splitting are those for blood pressure, cholesterol, and depression [36].

There are some important factors to consider when using this method to reduce costs. For example, not every pill or tablet should be split. Tablets that have been manufactured with scored lines are usually safe to split, but capsules or enteric-coated tablets should not be split or cut. A study on splitting antidepressant medications found that 41% of the split pills deviated from their ideal weight by 10%. While this is acceptable with some medications, it may greatly affect therapeutic levels in medications such as Coumadin and thyroid drugs [38]. Research conducted at Stanford University's Center for Research and Disease Prevention found 48 prescription mediations that are safe to cut or split [37]. Providers must also carefully consider whether the patient is a good candidate to perform the task. While pill splitters are available at most pharmacies, many patients with arthritis, poor eyesight, or memory problems may be unable to accomplish the task safely.

Seniors may be able to negotiate with their pharmacist to cut the pills for an additional charge and the pharmacist can check with the health care provider for the appropriate dosage change. Pharmacists can be an excellent resource for questions regarding the appropriateness of splitting medications. Senior citizens should be encouraged to discuss any questions about their medications with their pharmacist [39].

Patient education and advocacy

Patients need to be assertive in requesting generics from health care providers and pharmacists [40]. A study done by the Journal of the American Pharmacy Association found that most consumers were inclined to use generics, especially if their health care provider encouraged it. Seniors need to be educated not only on the value and safety of generics, but also on their rights to routinely request a generic substitution [29].

Many options for obtaining affordable medications are available to seniors, but a common problem is that senior citizens and the medical community are not aware of the existing resources. This presents an opportunity for nurses to act as patient advocates for senior citizens. The role of the registered nurse as a patient advocate is not a new one; patients trust nurses and the information provided by nurses. According to a press release by the International Council of Nurses, 90% of the public worldwide expressed confidence in nurses and acknowledged them as among the top professionals. The Council further stated that consumers trust the health education information provided by nurses, even if it may be contrary to another medical professional's [41].

Nurses have a responsibility to educate seniors on available health resources. Patricia Benner described nurses' role best when she said, "Being a good practitioner requires that we are moved by the patient's plight and that we respond to the patient as a person"[42].

Nurses providing care in offices, clinics, hospitals, and homes can help educate senior citizens and health care providers about the availability of resources that help with medication costs. In addition to contributing to patients' financial well-being, these interventions can enhance health status by promoting increased medication compliance.

References

[1] Steinman MA, Sands LP, Covinsky KE. Self-restriction of medications due to cost in seniors without prescription. J Gen Intern Med 2001;16:793–9.

[2] Kennedy J, Erb C. Prescription noncompliance due to cost amount adults with disabilities in the United States. Am J Public Health 2002;92(7):120–4.

[3] Allen I. Many seniors forced to skip prescription meds because of cost. Available at: http://www.cfah.org/hbns/newsrelease/prescription12-04-01. Accessed October 23, 2003.

[4] Cauchi R. States' Rx for drug cost. State Legis 2001;27(1):20–3.

[5] Hetzel L, Smith A. The 65 years and over population: 2000. US Census Bureau; October 2001: 1–8.

[6] O'Neill C, Hughes CM, Jamison J, et al. Cost of pharmacological care of the elderly: implications for healthcare resources. Drugs Aging 2003;20(4):253–61.

[7] Williams CM. Using medications appropriately in older adults. Am Fam Physician 2002; 66(10):1917–24.

[8] Gillette B. Battle over prescription drug intensifies. Mississippi Business Journal. August 14, 2000:26–7.

[9] Prescription drug bill expected to double over the next 10 years. Chemical Market Report. October 7, 2000;258(6):23.

[10] Anderson T. Taking a bite out of the sandwich generation (caring for elderly parents and children at the same time). USA Today [Magazine]. November 1999:1–2.

[11] Mojitaba R, Olfson M. Medicare costs, adherence, and health outcomes among Medicare beneficiaries. Health Aff 2003;22(4):220–5.

[12] Blustein J. Medicare and drug coverage: a women's health issue. Womens Health Issues 2000;10(2):47–53.

[13] Ganguli G. Consumers devise drug cost-cutting measures: medical and legal issues to consider. Health Care Manag 2003;22(3):275–81.

[14] Strengthening Medicare—President signs Medicare legislation [transcript]. Available at: http://www.whitehouse.gov/news/release/2003/12/20031208-2.html. Accessed January 15, 2004.

[15] Guthans S. Medicare reforms not effective until 2006. The Times-Picayune. January 15, 2004:1.

[16] Medicare Rights Center. Medicare Prescription Drug Cards. Available at: http://www.medicarerights.org/rxcards_faq.html. Accessed January 9, 2003.

[17] Proenza LR. The ABCs and D of Medicare. Available at: http://www.bankrate.com/brm/news/insurance/20040114al.asp. Accessed January 2004.

[18] Ritter J. Governor's study: Rx imports can save $91 million. Available at: http://www.suntimes.com/output/News/cst-nws-drugs27.html. Accessed October 10, 2003.

[19] Program to lower drug prices launched in Maine. Managed Care Weekly Digest. February 2, 2004, p. 104. Available at: http://www.NewsRx.com. Accessed February 10, 2004.

[20] Connony C. Illinois says import drugs could save state millions. Washington Post. October 22, 2003;A03.

[21] Zuckerman E. Rhode Island ponders buying drugs from Canada. Available at: http://news.Yahoo.com. Accessed January 14, 2004.

[22] American Association of Retired Persons. State-sponsored Rx drug discount program. Available at: http://www.AARP.com/yourmoney. Accessed November 3, 2003.

[23] Luckhart L. Seniors and prescription drugs. The Business Journal. May 21, 2004:7.

[24] Industry crack down on drug importation. Available at: http://www.newsday.com/news/nationworld/nation. Accessed July 14, 2004.

[25] Fisher M, Avorn J. Economic consequences of underused of generic drugs—evidence from Medicaid and implication for prescription drug benefit plans. Health Serv Res 2003;38(4): 1051–63.

[26] Wiebe C. Generic drugs offer relief from pain of rising drug cost. Medscape Money and Medicine 2002. Available at: http://www.medscape.com/viewarticle/438517. Accessed January 10, 2004.

[27] Edlin M. Flood of generic drugs causes a new wave of thrifty consumers. Managed Healthcare Executive 2003;4(5):40–1.

[28] Breitstein J. FDA touts generic message. Pharmaceutical Executive. October 2002; 22(10):130.

[29] Gaither C, Kirking D, Ascione F, et al. Consumers' views on generic medications. J Am Pharm Assoc 2001;31(5):729–36.

[30] These are the special drug discount programs recently introduced for senior citizens. Available at: http://www.seniorjournal.com/News/Medicare/03-23-02ListDrguDiscnts.htm. Accessed November 3, 2003.

[31] Volunteers in Healthcare. Are you looking for affordable medications? Available at: http://www.volunteersinhealthcare.org. Accessed November 3, 2003.

[32] Edwards D. Pharmacy discount card programs: catching up with the health market. Empl Benefits J 2002;27(3):42–3.

[33] Pfizer. Pfizer to launch comprehensive initiative expanding access to prescription medicines millions of Americans. Available at: http://www.pfizer.com/are/news_releases/A2004pr/mn_2004_0707.htm. Accessed July 14, 2004.

[34] Medicare. The official US Government site for people with Medicare. Available at: http://www.medicare.gov. Accessed November 3, 2003.

[35] American Association of Retired Persons. Available at: http://www.aarp.org. Accessed November 2, 2003.

[36] Cohen C, Cohen S. Potential savings from splitting newer antidepressant medications. CNS Drugs 2002;16(5):353–8.

[37] The Consumers Observation Post. It might be safe and cheaper to split your pills in half. Consumers Research Magazine 2002;85(10):7.

[38] Cut prescription drug costs by splitting pills–safely. Tuffs University Health and Nutrition Letter 2001;19(9):1.

[39] Splitting pills can mean big saving, but you need to do it right. Consum Rep Health 2000; 12(1):10.

[40] US Department of Defense Military Health System. Retirees. Available at: http://www.tricare.osd.mil/retirees. Accessed November 2, 2003.

[41] Bliss-Holtz J. Consumer trust—pass it on. Issues Compr Pediatr Nurs 2000;23:i–iii.

[42] Benner P. Enhancing patient advocacy and social ethics. Am J Crit Care 2003;12(4):374–5.

ELSEVIER
SAUNDERS

NURSING
CLINICS
OF NORTH AMERICA

Nurs Clin N Am 40 (2005) 63–75

Antibiotic Resistance

Maria A. Smith, DSN, RN, CCRN

School of Nursing, Middle Tennessee State University, 1500 Greenland Drive,
Box 81, Murfreesboro, TN 37132, USA

Concerns about the source and mechanism of the spread of disease are not new societal issues. Ancient records revealed that the Egyptians and Chinese used asepsis for wounds and injuries. Hippocrates burned aromatic wood in the streets of Athens in an attempt to stop the plague. In the early 1800s, various methods for safely preserving food for long sea voyages were developed. The fact that cleanliness was linked to disease was also a realization of this era. The mid-1800s saw the development of pasteurization to prevent souring of milk by controlling microorganisms. In the late 1800s, scientifically based procedures for dry heat and steam sterilization were developed. These events laid the foundation for management of microorganism invasion of the body with oils, herbs and medications.

The development of penicillin in 1929 was a major breakthrough in microorganism management, but industrialization of the antibiotic was not realized until World War II (1939–1945). Penicillin's mode of action was by preventing cross-linking of small peptide chains in peptidoglycan, which was the main polymer of bacteria. Penicillin G was derived from the culture filtrate *Penicillium notatum* or *P chrysogenum.* Penicillin was effective against gram-positive bacteria. This antibiotic served as a valuable tool in the treatment of war wounds infected with *Staphylococcus.* Natural penicillins could be chemically modified by adding acyl groups, which conferred new properties and resulted in a semisynthetic penicillin (eg, ampicillin and oxacillin). These semisynthetic penicillins were resistant to stomach acids and offered a degree of resistance to penicillinase, a penicillin-destroying enzyme. The remarkable success of penicillin led to the discovery of other antibiotics such as streptomycin, which was effective against gram-negative bacteria (Table 1).

Breakthroughs in research gave practitioners an arsenal of antibiotics to use against bacteria that produce numerous illnesses. More antibiotics with

E-mail address: massmith@mtsu.edu

0029-6465/05/$ - see front matter © 2005 Elsevier Inc. All rights reserved.
doi:10.1016/j.cnur.2004.08.006   *nursing.theclinics.com*

Table 1
Antibiotic examples

Antibiotic	Bacterial activity affected	Site of action
Bacitracin	Gram-positive	Wall synthesis
Cephalosporin	Broad spectrum	Wall synthesis
Erythromycin	Gram-positive	Protein synthesis
Gentamycin	Broad spectrum	Protein synthesis
Neomycin	Broad spectrum	Protein synthesis
Penicillin	Gram-positive	Wall synthesis
Streptomycin	Gram-negative	Protein synthesis
Tetracycline	Broad spectrum	Protein synthesis
Vancomycin	Gram-positive	Protein synthesis

expanded modes of action led to indiscriminate use for illnesses, regardless of whether they were bacterial or nonbacterial. For instance, most upper respiratory infections are viral in nature, but every year, millions of antibiotic prescriptions are written for viral infections because of patient demand, physician time constraints, and diagnostic uncertainty. However, viruses do not respond to antibiotic treatment. According to the Centers for Disease Control and Prevention (CDC), antibiotic use for upper respiratory infections may not be warranted (Table 2) [1].

Use of antibiotics in humans was not the only mechanism that contributed to antibiotic resistance [2]. Antibiotic use in animals for therapeutic management related to food production and disease prevention also promoted antibiotic resistance in humans. Low doses of antibiotics administered to food-producing animals can result in bacterial resistance in or near livestock. This practice elevates the potential for resistant bacterial strains to cross species, especially livestock imported from countries where antibiotic use is indiscriminate (ie, antibiotics may be obtained and administered to livestock without specific guidelines).

Misuse and abuse has led to antibiotic resistance through a process of natural selection [3,4]. When antibiotics are administered to treat bacterial invasion, the microorganisms that are more susceptible die. The remaining bacteria are resistant. These microorganisms can pass on resistance in one of two ways: (1) by replication through genes to their offspring, or (2) by conjugation where gene-carrying plasmids jump from one organism to another. It is important to be aware of this naturally occurring phenomenon when considering treatment options [5].

Drug access also affects antibiotic resistance. Individuals who have insurance are afforded an option to obtain diagnosis and treatment from a health care professional. Those with limited resources resort to self-diagnosis and treatment with poor-quality drugs or borrowed portions of antibiotics from an associate. These circumstances potentiate antibiotic resistance through more rapid selection of resistant organisms.

Table 2
Recommended antibiotic use for upper respiratory infections

Diagnosis	Antibiotic recommendation
Otitis media with effusion (OME)	Not for initial treatment of OME. May be indicated if bilateral effusions persist for 3 months or more.
Acute otitis media (AOM)	Consider antibiotics for greater than 3 documented episodes in 6 months (or greater than 4 in 12 months)
Rhinitis	Not indicated for viral rhinosinusitis or mucopurulent rhinitis unless it persists without improvement for greater than 10–14 days.
Sinusitis	Initial antibiotic treatment with narrow spectrum agent may be warranted in the presence of symptoms of acute sinus infection.
Pharyngitis	Not in the absence of group A streptococcal infection. Penicillin drug of choice for treatment of group A streptococcal pharyngitis.
Bronchitis	Not recommended in well-appearing individuals with cough lesser than 10–14 days and no physical signs of pneumonia.
Pertussis	May be warranted for cough greater than 10 days in children with underlying chronic pulmonary disease.
Flu	Not recommended.
Viral upper respiratory infection (URI)	Not recommended even in the presence of mucous changes to green or yellow.

Counterfeit drugs also directly contribute to antibiotic resistance. As health care costs increase, people seek ways to manage expenses. One mechanism is to reduce monies spent on prescription medications. In the past 5 years, the use of internet-based, non–United States pharmacies to obtain drugs has flourished. Between 1992 and 1994, the World Health Organization (WHO) discovered that of the counterfeiting cases identified, 70% were not based in the United States. According to the WHO inquiry, 51% of counterfeit drugs carried no active ingredients, 17% contained incorrect ingredients, and 11% contained less than the recommended concentration of active ingredients [6]. Some medications actually contained poisons that could result in severe disability or death. Only 4% of counterfeit drugs were equal to their authentic counterpart in quality [6].

Scope of the problem

Half of the 100 million antibiotic prescriptions written annually in office-based health care settings are unnecessary because they are for infections of viral origin [7]. Because of increased use of antibiotics, infections such as gonorrhea and childhood ear infections that previously responded to cheaper first-line antibiotics have become increasingly difficult to treat. As a result, infections transition from organ confinement to generalized sepsis.

Sepsis affects approximately 750,000 people in the United States, resulting in the death of approximately 225,000 individuals per year. Approximately 2 million people get hospital-acquired infections, resulting in 90,000 deaths [8]. More than 70% of bacteria that cause hospital-acquired infections are resistant to first-line antibiotics [9]. When infections fail to respond to first-line antibiotics, treatment must resort to second- and third-line drugs. These drugs can be 10 to 100 times more expensive, with more severe and toxic side effects. For some individuals, alternate medications can be cost prohibitive. Alternative means of treatment may result in more severe forms of the illness for which treatment was originally sought or even death. Individuals for whom cost does not pose an impediment to treatment still run the risk of encountering antibiotic resistance, which could mean additional visits to a health care provider, and the use of more potent and potentially toxic drugs.

This era of emerging antibiotic resistance has resulted in the identification of organisms resistant to drugs such as vancomycin, methicillin, and penicillin. Though numerous antibiotic-resistant types of bacteria exist, one of the most well known is methicillin-resistant *Staphylococcus aureus* (MRSA). Other types are listed in Box 1.

Antibiotic resistance and globalization

International travel has made the world borderless to microorganism invasion [10]. Organisms that originate on one continent can be spread worldwide in a few hours. Medications also freely cross borders. Travelers can retrieve antibiotics that have various degrees of effectiveness from countries with poor pharmacologic development guidelines.

Various departments, which often fail to coordinate management of disease identification and intervention, govern health care in developing countries. Poor interdepartmental communication permits diseases to reach various epidemic stages before government and health care intervention

---

Box 1. Antibiotic resistant organisms

Extended-spectrum β-lactamases (ESBLs)
Vancomycin-resistant *Enterococcus* (VRE)
Vancomycin-intermediate *Staphylococcus aureus* (VISA)
Vancomycin-resistant *Staphylococcus aureus* (VRSA)
Methicillin-resistant *S aureus* (MRSA)
Drug-resistant *Streptococcus pneumoniae* (DRSP)
Methicillin-susceptible *S aureus* (MSSA)
Penicillin-resistant *S pneumoniae* (PRSP)

occur. Disease management in these countries is affected by the lack of governmental recognition regarding the severity of diseases that require intervention for the health of the general population. Failure to implement timely and effective guidelines also promotes the spread of antibiotic resistance.

Antibiotic resistant types

Methicillin-resistant Staphylococcus aureus

S aureus is often found in 20% to 30% of the nasal mucosa of healthy individuals. It can also be identified on the external skin surface. *S aureus* that is resistant to methicillin is referred to as methicillin-resistant *S aureus* (MRSA). MRSA strains that occur in epidemic proportions are referred to as EMRSA. The number of specific laboratory techniques that were used to distinguish EMRSA type is attached to the abbreviation to give specificity to the epidemic (eg, EMRSA-16).

S aureus is a leading cause of nosocomial infection in the United States. MRSA poses serious challenges to the treatment of hospital-acquired infections. MRSA carries a uniquely effective resistance mechanism that protects the pathogen against all members of the β-lactam family of antibiotics [11].

Because *Staphylococcus* colonies (positive cultures found in the absence of signs or symptoms of infection) are found mostly in the nasal mucosa, autoinfection is responsible for many infections that occur in health care and community settings. Airborne transmission or transmission by way of fomite (ie, an inanimate object) is rare.

MRSA is a contact organism. Health care workers can be significant facilitators of the spread of the organism. Transmission can occur if proper handwashing and glove-wearing procedures are not routinely practiced. Gowns should also be worn if there is the potential for contamination by way of suppurative lesions.

Vancomycin-intermediate Staphylococcus aureus/*Vancomycin-resistant* Staphylococcus aureus

Vancomycin-intermediate *S aureus* (VISA) and vancomycin-resistant *S aureus* (VRSA) are specific forms of *S aureus* that are resistant to the medication vancomycin. The specific forms of *S aureus* that are classified as VISA or VRSA are identified by using laboratory tests that determine the amount of vancomycin required to prohibit organism growth. Test results may be expressed as a minimum inhibitory concentration (MIC). The MIC identifies the minimum amount of medication required to inhibit growth in a test tube. If the MIC for vancomycin is 8 to 16 µg/mL, the staphylococcal infection is classified as VISA. If the MIC is elevated to over 32 µg/mL, the staphylococcal infection is classified as VRSA.

VISA and VRSA infections are not common occurrences. Cases have been reported in Michigan, New Jersey, New York, Illinois, Nevada, and Pennsylvania where the infections occurred in individuals who were compromised by underlying health conditions, previous infections with MRSA, or exposure to vancomycin and other antibiotics.

Drug-resistant Streptococcus pneumoniae

Streptococcal pneumonia is a leading cause of illness and death. Clinical features include pneumonia, otitis media, sinusitis, and meningitis. These diseases account for varying degrees of hearing loss and neurologic sequelae. Streptococcal pneumonia can be spread through person-to-person contact and respiratory droplets. Annually, streptococcal pneumonia accounts for approximately 100,000 to 135,000 hospitalized cases of pneumonia, 6 million cases of otitis media, and 60,000 cases of invasive disease, including 3300 cases of meningitis [12]. The pneumococcal conjugate vaccine for children is reducing these numbers.

Streptococcus pneumoniae infections that are resistant to one or more antibiotics are referred to as drug-resistant *S pneumoniae* (DRSP). There are seven identified serotypes that account for most cases of DRSP. These subtypes are 6A, 6B, 9V, 14, 19A, 19F, and 23F. Approximately 40% of infections result from pneumococci resistant to at least one antibiotic and 15% of pneumococcal infections are resistant to three or more drugs.

Strategies to prevent the spread of DRSP include hand-management techniques (eg, handwashing and glove wearing) and patient education. Environmental management of airborne droplets, including covering the mouth and nose while sneezing and coughing, and proper disposal of contaminated material, are important. Vaccination against pneumococcal diseases is recommended for high-risk children (over 2 years of age) and individuals 65 years of age or older.

Mechanisms of resistance to current antibiotic agents

Resistance to β-lactams (eg, penicillins) can occur as a result of (1) inactivation of antibiotics by β-lactamase, (2) modification of target penicillin-binding proteins (PBPs), (3) impaired penetration of a drug to target PBPs, or (4) the presence of an efflux pump. The most common mechanism of resistance is β-lactamase production. β-lactamases are produced by bacteria such as *S aureus*, *E coli*, and *Pseudomonas aeruginosa*. Alteration in target PBPs is responsible for staphylococci resistance to methicillin and pneumococci resistance to penicillin. The PBPs produced by these organisms have a low affinity for binding β-lactam antibiotics. Resistance caused by impaired penetration of antibiotics to target PBPs occurs only in gram-negative bacteria, because of the impermeability of the outer membrane. Gram-negative bacteria may also produce an efflux pump that transports some β-lactam antibiotics back across the outer cell.

Resistance to vancomycin is directly related to its mechanism of action, which involves the inhibition of cell wall synthesis. Vancomycin inhibits peptidoglycan biosynthesis through modification of the D-Ala-D-Ala binding site of the peptidoglycan building block [13]. The terminal D-Ala is replaced by D-Lactate. This alteration results in the loss of a critical hydrogen bond, decreased affinity binding, and the loss of vancomycin activity.

Resistance to tetracyclines occurs as a result of (1) enzymatic inactivation, (2) reduced intracellular drug accumulation due to impaired influx or increased efflux by transport protein pump, or (3) ribosome protection due to production of proteins that interfere with binding of tetracycline to the ribosome. The protein pump is encoded. Efflux pump production results in protein encoding, which may be transmitted through transduction or conjugation. The efflux pump can cause resistance to multiple drugs (eg, sulfonamides and aminoglycosides).

Resistance to erythromycin occurs as a result of (1) production of starases that hydrolyze macrolides, (2) active reflux or reduced permeability of the cell membrane, and (3) modification of the ribosomal binding site through chromosomal mutation and production of constitutive methylase. Constitutive methylase production is also responsible for resistance to such drugs as clindamycin.

New antibiotic agents

Nosocomial infections caused by gram-positive cocci have exceeded those caused by gram-negative bacilli. In response to this increasing threat, newer antibiotic agents are being developed to combat gram-positive cocci. There are several new drugs on the horizon to fight infections caused by gram-positive organisms. These drugs include dalbavancin, daptomycin, oritavancin (in development), ramoplanin (in development), and telithromycin.

Dalbavancin is a once-weekly injectable antibiotic. It will be active against skin infections involving resistant pathogens such as MRSA. In Phase II clinical trials, dalbavancin was compared with vancomycin, a current treatment. Preliminary results revealed higher clinical and microbiologic response rates in patients treated with dalbavancin. In November 2003, this drug was in Phase III clinical trials. Drugs go through three stages of clinical trials before a company applies with the US Food and Drug Administration (FDA) to market it [14]. The submission of the new drug application (NDA) for dalbavancin is anticipated later in 2004.

Daptomycin was approved by the FDA in September 2003 and was included in a new classification of antibiotics known as lipopeptides, which are used to treat complicated skin and skin structure infections caused by gram-positive bacteria, including MRSA and methicillin-susceptible *S aureus* [15]. The drug is designed to be administered intravenously once every 24 hours for 7 to 14 days. Daptomycin acts by binding to bacterial membranes and causing rapid depolarization of the membrane potential. Membrane potential loss leads to inhibition of DNA, RNA, and protein synthesis, which ultimately results in bacterial cell death. Dose adjustment is required in patients who have renal impairment.

Oritavancin is a second-generation glycopeptide that has bactericidal activity. It will be effective against gram-positive bacteria including those resistant to vancomycin. This drug is pending approval by the FDA. The NDA for oritavancin is expected to be filed in early 2005.

Ramoplanin is the first in a new class of antimicrobials known as glycolipodepsipeptides. Clinical trials have shown that Ramoplanin has excellent in vitro activity against both vancomycin-resistant *Enterococcus faecium* and *E faecalis*. It is orally administered and is not absorbed systemically. It is designed to reduce antibiotic resistance through its mechanism of action. Ramoplanin works by attaching itself to an essential sugar within the cell wall, which would require the cell to go through multiple evolutionary steps and change its mechanism for development of the cell membrane to develop resistance. This orally administered antibiotic is 2 to 10 times more active than vancomycin against some gram-positive bacteria. Ramoplanin is currently in a Phase III clinical trial for the prevention of bloodstream infections caused by vancomycin-resistant Enterococci (VRE) and a Phase II clinical trial for the treatment of *Clostridium* difficile-associated diarrhea [16].

Telithromycin is a ketolide that was approved by the FDA in January 2003. It is the first ketolide to be awarded approvable status for clinical use. Ketolides are chemically different macrolide derivatives. A key action of telithromycin is against infections caused by multi–drug-resistant *S pneumoniae* [17]. It was approved for the treatment of community-acquired pneumonia, acute exacerbations of chronic bronchitis, and acute bacterial sinusitis. Currently, this daily dosed antibiotic only has an oral mode of administration. Therapy duration ranges from 5 days for respiratory infections to up to 10 days for community-acquired pneumonia. The most commonly reported side effects are diarrhea and nausea [18].

Quinupristin-dalfopristin is a new bacteriocidal medication. This drug is active against Staphylococci and *E faecium*, but not against *E fecalis*. It must be given through a central line because of its vein sclerosis property. Dose adjustment is required in patients who have hepatic failure. Though well-tolerated, the drug may cause myalgias and arthralgias. Quinupristin-dalfopristin should be administered with caution to patients who are receiving other drugs metabolized by the hepatic cytochrome p450 system because of the occurrence of drug interactions.

Linezolid is a new bacteriostatic agent against Staphylococci and Enterococci. This drug is active against MRSA and VRE. It is available intravenously and orally and is well-tolerated. Side effects of Linezolid include granulocytopenia and thrombocytopenia (usually during the second week of therapy). Pseudoephedrine and serum-uptake inhibitors should be administered with caution in patients receiving Linezolid, because it is a weak monamine oxidase inhibitor.

The evolving arsenal of new medications presents opportunities and challenges in the management of antibiotic-resistant bacteria by health care providers. Many drugs have been approved within the past 2 years and require continued evaluation for the development of new side effects. Clinicians must remain current and continue to update their database of antibiotics for patient management.

Action plan for antibiotic resistance

The unnecessary use of systemic antibacterials has been a leading cause for the rise in antibiotic resistance in the past 5 to 10 years. This rise has occurred in both hospital and community-acquired infections. First steps to addressing the problem of antibiotic resistance are awareness and education of health care providers and the public. Education of health care providers about the hazards of prescribing antibiotics for illnesses that are non-bacterial will go a long way in decreasing the prevalence, and slowing the spread, of antibiotic resistance.

In February 2003, the FDA announced new labeling requirements for all systemic antibacterial drug products intended for human use in an effort to address the growing development of antibiotic-resistant bacteria [19]. Statements regarding proper usage of antibiotics to reduce the development of antibiotic resistance were recommended for inclusion. This government intervention was aimed at reducing inappropriate and indiscriminate use of antibiotics in children and adults for treatment of ear infections and chronic coughs.

Hand hygiene is important in the management of microbes in hospital and community settings [20]. Proper handwashing, and improved adherence to wearing gloves and using alcohol-based rubs when appropriate, have been shown to reduce antimicrobial transmission and overall infection rates.

Handwashing remains a first line of defense against the spread of microorganisms. Proper handwashing includes the use of soap and water in cooperation with the specific technique of using friction over an ample amount of time. This promotes the cleaning of all hand surfaces. Gloves can prevent hand contamination by 70% to 80% and should be worn as a protective barrier and to prevent cross contamination when suppurative lesions are present. Hands should always be washed when gloves are removed [20]. Nurses have a direct responsibility to address antibiotic-resistance procedures in all settings (Fig. 1).

Limiting antibiotic use is another strategy to address antibiotic resistance. One starting point is to use short-course antibiotic therapy (3 days). This

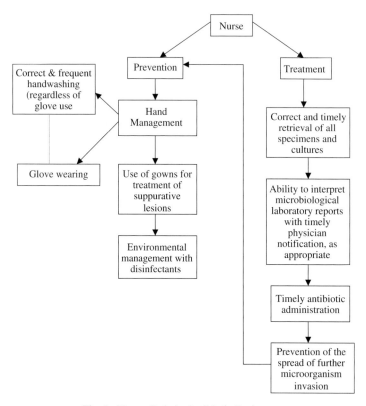

Fig. 1. Nurses Role in Antibiotic Resistance.

technique has proven to decrease colonization or superinfection with resistant organisms within intensive care units in patients at low risk for pneumonia and in patients who have new infiltrates [21,22]. Implementation of these antibiotics should be for specific pathogens identified from diagnostic testing and culture analysis.

Once-daily aminoglycoside dosing for patients may also reduce the incidence of antibiotic resistance [23,24]. Once-daily dosing minimizes the potential for ototoxicity and nephrotoxicity, allows for maximal antibiotic efficacy, and takes advantage of concentration-dependent killing of micro-organisms. Administration of medication in once-daily doses also reduces medication error potential by using a consistent dose that is not based on aminoglycoside levels. This strategy reduces health care costs by eliminating multiple medication dose preparations by the pharmacy and reducing the frequency of medication administration by nurses.

Programs have been developed to address the issue of antibiotic resistance. Criteria-based antibiotic guides are being developed by in-dependent health care agencies at the state and federal levels. Surveillance is multileveled as well. The National Antimicrobial Resistance Monitoring

Table 3
National antimicrobial resistance monitoring system data reporting for antibiotic resistance monitoring

Number of agencies		
State	Local	Reporting process
10	0	First clinical *Campylobacter* isolate received each week
50	4	Every twentieth *E coli* O157:H7 case
10	0	Twenty human enterococcal isolates each week
50	4	Every twentieth non-typhi *Salmonella* case
50	4	Every twentieth *Shigella* case

Abbreviations: NARMS, National antimicrobial resistance monitoring system.

System (NARMS) for enteric bacteria was established in 1996. NARMS evolved within the framework of the Centers for Disease Control and Emerging Infections Program's Epidemiology and Laboratory Capacity Program and the Foodborne Diseases Active Surveillance Network (FoodNet). This central antimicrobial-resistance monitoring program facilitates data collection and trend analysis for identification of emerging resistance. Currently NARMS monitors antibiotic resistance in diseases caused by *Campylobacter*, *E coli* 0157, *Enterococcus*, non-Typhi *Salmonella*, *Salmonella typhi*, and *Shigella* (Table 3).

Summary

Resistance to antibiotics is economically and physiologically costly [25]. Control of antibiotic resistance will require aggressive implementation of numerous strategies [26]. Ongoing surveillance is needed to monitor known antibiotic types and to be able to identify the development of other potential types. Early intervention is needed to combat the rising rate of resistance. Persistent use of hygiene measures and controlled use of antibiotics will limit the spread of antibiotic resistance.

Health care providers need to monitor adherence to control measures. Hand and environmental control measures remain a critical component of staff education activities. Active management of infections with non-pharmacologic treatments should be promoted. Motivational campaigns will reinforce positive infection control behaviors. Consistent surveillance of antibiotic use will help fulfill the CDC directive to combat antibiotic resistance and keep the population healthy.

References

[1] Dowell SF, Marcy SM, Phillips WR, Gerber MA, Schwartz B. Principles of judicious use of antimicrobial agents for pediatric upper respiratory tract infections. Pediatrics 1998; 101(Suppl 1):163–5. Available at: http://www.cdc.gov/drugresistance/community/technical.htm. Accessed January 17, 2004.

[2] Anderson AD, Nelson JM, Rossiter S, Angulo FJ. Public health consequences of use of antimicrobial agents in food animals in the United States. Microb Drug Resist 2003; 9(4):373–9. Available at: http://www.cdc.gov/narms/pub/publications/a_anderson.pdf. Accessed December 22, 2003.

[3] Skirble R. Abuse, overuse of antibiotics creates public health crisis. VOA News 2003;17:13. Available at: http://www.VOANews.com. Accessed December 10, 2003.

[4] Stratton CW. Dead bugs don't mutate: susceptibility issues in the emergence of bacterial resistance. Emerg Infect Dis [serial online] 2003 Jan. Available at: http://www.cdc.gov/ncidod/EID/vol19no1/02-0175.htm. Accessed January 3, 2004.

[5] Workman ML. The cellular basis of bacterial infection. Crit Care Nurs Clin North Am 2003; 15(1):1–11.

[6] World Health Organization. Factors contributing to resistance. Infectious Disease Report. 2000. Available at: http://www.who.int/infectious-disease-report/2000/ch3.htm. Accessed December 1, 2003.

[7] Centers for Disease Control and Prevention. Antibiotic resistance: technical information. Available at: http://www.cdc.gov/drugresistance/community/technical.htm. Accessed January 17, 2004.

[8] Centers for Disease Control and Prevention. Department of Health and Human Services. Available at: http://www.cdc.gov. Accessed December 2, 2003.

[9] Bren L. Battle of the bugs: fighting antibiotic resistance. FDA Magazine. Vol. 36, No. 4. July–August 2002. Available at: http://www.fda.gov/fdac/features/2002/402_bugs.html. Accessed November 17, 2003.

[10] Sanchez IS, Ramirez M, Troni H, Abecassis M, Padua M, Tomasz A, et al. Evidence for the geographic spread of a methicillin-resistant Staphylococcus-aureus clone between Portugal and Spain. J Clin Microbiol 1995;33(5):1243–6.

[11] Crisóstomo MI, Westh H, Tomasz A, Chung M, Oliveira DC, deLencaste H. The evolution of methicillin resistant Staphylococcus aureus: similarity of genetic backgrounds in historically early methicillin-susceptible and -resistant isolates and contemporary epidemic clones. Proc Natl Acad Sci USA 1998;(17):9865–70.

[12] Centers for Disease Control and Prevention. Drug-resistant Streptococcus pneumonia disease. Available at: http://www.cdc.gov/ncidod/dbmd/diseaseinfo/drugresistreppneum_t. htm. Accessed January 3, 2004.

[13] Walsh C. Molecular mechanisms that confer antibacterial drug resistance. Nature 2001;406: 775–81.

[14] Centers for Disease Control and Prevention. The new drug development process: steps from test tube to new drug application review. Available at http://www.fda.gov/cder/handbook/develop.htm. Accessed April 2, 2004.

[15] Food and Drug Administration. FDA Drug Approvals List. Available at: http://www.fda.gov/cder/foi/label/2003/21572_cubicin_lbl.pdf. Accessed January 8, 2004.

[16] Genome Therapeutics Corporation. Ramoplanin: a novel antibiotic for serious bacterial infections. Available at http://www.genomecorp.com//programs/pdf/RamoplaninBackgrounder.pdf. Accessed April 2, 2004.

[17] Bearden DT, Neuhauser MM, Garey KW. Telithromycin: an oral ketolide for respiratory infections. Pharmacotherapy 2001;21(10):1204–22.

[18] Uriarte SM, Molestina RE, Miller RD, Bernabo J, Farinati A, Eiguchi K, et al. Effect of macrolide antibiotics on human endothelial cells activated by Chlamydia pneumonia infection and tumor necrosis factor. J Infect Dis 2002;185:1631–6.

[19] Department of Health and Human Services. Food and Drug Administration. Labeling requirements for systemic and antibacterial drug products intended for human use. Final rule. 2003; 21CFR Part 201. Available at: http://www.fda.gov/OHRMS/DOCKETS/98fr/00n-1463-nfr00001.pdf.

[20] Centers for Disease Control and Prevention. Hand hygiene guidelines fact sheet. Available at: http://www.cdc.gov/od/oc/media/pressrel/fs021025.htm. Accessed December 22, 2003.

[21] Singh N, Rogers P, Atwood CW, Wagener MM, Yu VL. Short course empiric antibiotic therapy for patients with pulmonary infiltrates in the intensive care unit. A proposed solution for indiscriminate antibiotic prescription. A J Respir Crit Care Med 2000;162(2 Pt 1):505–11.

[22] Steinberg I. Clinical choices of antibiotics: Judging judicious use. Am J Manage Care 2000;6(23)(Suppl):S1178–88, S1241–2.

[23] Timm E. Infection: antibiotics. Once daily aminoglycoside dosing in ICU patients. Presented at Program and Abstracts of the 32nd Critical Care Congress; San Antonio, January 28– February 2, 2003.

[24] Kolef MH. Is there a role for antibiotic cycling in the intensive care unit? Crit Care Med 2001; 29(Suppl 4):N135–42.

[25] Sommers BD. Economics of antibiotic resistance. Crit Care Nurs Clinic North Am 2003; 15(1):89–96.

[26] Weinstein RA, Kabins SA. Strategies for prevention and control of multiple-drug resistant nosocomial infections. Am J Med 1981;70:449–54.

ELSEVIER
SAUNDERS

NURSING
CLINICS
OF NORTH AMERICA

Nurs Clin N Am 40 (2005) 77–94

Innovations in Antineoplastic Therapy

Roberta Kaplow, RN, PhD, CCNS, CCRN

Nell Hodgson Woodruff School of Nursing, Emory University, Atlanta, GA, USA

Innovations in the treatment of cancer are developed on a regular basis. The US Food and Drug Administration (FDA) frequently makes announcements about agents that are approved for either clinical trials or clinician use as part of the arsenal against cancer. Ongoing research in the basic sciences has led to an enhanced understanding of cancer. This knowledge has resulted in new key scientific advances in combating the disease.

This article reviews the antineoplastic therapies that have received FDA approval within the past 3 years. Some of the agents may not be new but have been granted approval for a new indication or mode of administration. Categories of agents include chemotherapy, biotherapy, and hormonal therapies. A brief description of the mechanism of action, clinical indications, and reported adverse effects is provided. Select therapies currently in the pipeline are also mentioned. Some of these latter agents are in the early stages of exploration to determine their value, and may be considered part of standard therapy in the future. A summary of all of the newly approved agents appears in Table 1.

Innovations in chemotherapy

Oxaliplatin (Eloxatin)

Oxaliplatin is a new platinum-based chemotherapeutic agent that was approved by the FDA in August 2002 [1]. It is approved for use with 5-fluorouracil (5-FU) and leucovorin (LV), a combination that is considered first-line therapy for the treatment of patients who have metastatic colorectal cancer, or recurrent or progressive disease during or within 6 months after completion of the 5-FU/LV and irinotecan combination bolus [2].

Oxaliplatin is a cell cycle non-specific alkylating agent. It is effective against cancer because of its ability to block DNA replication and transcription. It works synergistically with 5-FU.

E-mail address: rkaplow@emory.edu

doi:10.1016/j.cnur.2004.08.007   *nursing.theclinics.com*

Table 1
Summary of innovations in antineoplastic therapies

Category	Generic (trade) name	Date approved	Primary or new indication
Chemotherapy	Oxaliplatin (Eloxatin)	8/02	For use in combination with 5-fluorouracil (5-FU) and leucovorin (LV), for the treatment of patients who have metastatic colorectal cancer or recurrent or progressive disease during or within 6 months of completion of combination bolus 5-FU/LV and irinotecan
Chemotherapy	Fludarabine phosphate (Fludara)	12/01	For treatment of B-cell chronic lymphocytic leukemia (CLL) in patients who have not responded to or whose disease has progressed during treatment with at least one standard regimen that contains an alkylating agent
Chemotherapy	Polifeprosan 20 with carmustine implant (Gliadel) wafer	2/03	Used in newly diagnosed patients who have high-grade malignant glioma as an adjunct to surgery and radiation therapy. It had been previously approved in 1997 as an adjunct to treatment for another type of brain tumor known as glioblastoma multiforme brain tumors
Chemotherapy	Capecitabine (Xeloda)	9/01	Used as part of combination therapy with docetaxel (Taxotere) for treating patients who have metastatic breast cancer whose cancer has progressed after treatment with an anthracycline
Chemotherapy	Docetaxel (Taxotere)	11/02	For patients who have advanced breast cancer that has progressed despite treatment with standard cancer treatment, such as doxorubicin. In 2002, it was approved for first-line treatment in combination with cisplatin for treatment of unresectable, locally advanced or metastatic non-small cell lung cancer
Biotherapy	Ibritumomab tiuxetan (Zevalin)	2/02	As part of the treatment for relapsed or refractory low-grade follicular or transformed B-cell non-Hodgkin's lymphoma
Biotherapy	Tositumomab and iodine 131 tositumomab (Bexxar)	6/03	For the treatment of CD20 positive follicular non-Hodgkin's lymphoma

Biotherapy	Alemtuzumab (Campath)	8/01	For the treatment of chronic lymphocytic leukemia. Originally approved in 2001 for treatment of B-cell CLL in patients who have been treated with alkylating agents and have failed treatment with fludarabine
Biotherapy	Imatinib mesylate (Gleevac)	12/03	For treatment of patients who have Philadelphia chromosome positive chronic myeloid leukemia in blast crisis
Biotherapy	Bortezomib (Velcade)	6/03	For treatment of patients who have multiple myeloma, received at least 2 prior therapies, and have disease progression since the last therapy
Biotherapy	Gemtuzumab ozogomicin (Mylotarg)	5/00	For the treatment of patients 60 years or over who have CD33 positive acute myeloid leukemia that has relapsed for the first time and who are poor candidates for cytotoxic therapy
Biotherapy	Arsenic Trioxide (Trsenox)	9/00	For the treatment of patients with acute promyelocytic leukemia (APL) who have not responded to, or relapsed following, the use of the first-line therapy all trans-retinoic acid and chemotherapy with anthracyclines
Biotherapy	Bevacizumab (Avastin)	2/04	As a first-line treatment of patients who have metastatic colorectal cancer
Biotherapy	Cetuximab (Erbitux)	2/04	To treat patients who have metastatic colorectal cancer, used either in combination with irinotecan or as a single-agent therapy
Biotherapy	Gefitinib (Iressa)	5/03	For single-agent therapy of locally advanced or metastatic NSCLC that has progressed despite treatment with other chemotherapy, specifically platinum-based agents and docetaxel
Hormonal therapy	Anastrazole (Arimidex)	9/02	As adjuvant (supplementary) treatment for postmenopausal women who have locally advanced or metastatic breast cancer
Hormonal therapy	Exemestane (Aromasin)	11/03	For postmenopausal women for whom tamoxifen has stopped working

(continued on next page)

Table 1 (*continued*)

Category	Generic (trade) name	Date approved	Primary or new indication
Hormonal therapy	Letrozole (Femera)	1/01	Initially approved for women who have breast cancer and did not respond to antiestrogen therapy. It is now a first line therapy for postmenopausal women who have locally advanced or metastatic breast cancer
Hormonal therapy	Fulvestrant (Faslodex)	4/02	For the treatment of hormone receptor positive metastatic breast cancer in postmenopausal women who have disease progression following antiestrogen therapy (eg, tamoxifen)
Hormonal therapy	Leuprolide (Eligard)	2/03	Initially approved for treatment of prostate cancer. In 2002, a sustained release version was approved, thereby changing the dosing frequency from every month to every 3 months. Most recently, it was approved for the palliative treatment of advanced prostate cancer
Hormonal therapy	Abrelix (Plenaxis)	11/03	For the treatment of symptoms of advanced prostate cancer for which there are no other therapeutic options

The most frequently reported adverse events when oxaliplatin is used in combination with 5-FU/LV infusions include fatigue, diarrhea, abdominal pain, stomatitis (ie, inflammation of the mouth), dyspnea, nausea, and vomiting. Patients may also develop anemia, leukopenia, neutropenia, and thrombocytopenia. Pulmonary toxicity may also occur in patients who have received oxaliplatin. A small percentage of patients also report specific types of peripheral sensory neuropathies, including pharyngolaryngeal dysesthesia characterized by sensations of "swallowing glass" upon exposure to cold air or liquids following treatment, and the sensation of pain, numbness, or tingling when hands or feet come in contact with cold (eg, a cold drinking vessel or floor, respectively) [2,3].

Fludarabine phosphate (Fludara)

Fludarabine was approved by the FDA in December 2001 for treatment of B-cell chronic lymphocytic leukemia (CLL) in patients who have not responded to, or whose disease has progressed during, treatment with at least one standard regimen that contains an alkylating agent. Fludarabine is an antimetabolite that shortens the lifespan of existing leukemic cells and inhibits DNA synthesis so that new leukemia cells cannot grow [3].

The most common side effects reported with fludarabine are myelosuppression, fever, chills, infection, nausea, and vomiting. Other adverse events include malaise, fatigue, anorexia, weakness, agitation, confusion, visual disturbances, gastrointestinal bleeding, and stomatitis. Pneumonia, a frequently occurring infection in patients with CLL, has also been reported in patients who are being treated with fludarabine. Acute tumor lysis syndrome has been observed in patients who have large tumor burdens. Instances of autoimmune hemolytic anemia have also been described [4].

Polifeprosan 20 with carmustine implant (Gliadel) wafer

The FDA approved the polifeprosan 20 with carmustine wafer in February 2003 for use in newly diagnosed patients with high-grade malignant glioma (a type of brain tumor) as an adjunct to surgery and radiation therapy. It was previously approved in 1997 as an adjunct to treatment for another type of brain tumor known as glioblastoma multiforme brain tumors [2].

The polifeprosan 20 with carmustine wafer is approximately the size of a dime. It slowly delivers chemotherapy directly to the tumor, bypassing the blood-brain-barrier. This action helps minimize the systemic side effects associated with traditional chemotherapy. The wafer is placed in the cavity that is created when the brain tumor is resected and the chemotherapy is delivered directly to the tumor site [2,3].

Reported adverse effects of the polifeprosan 20 with carmustine wafer include seizures, brain hemorrhage, brain cyst, cerebral edema, wound infection, and brain abscess. These events may be attributed either to the surgery, the wafer placement, or both [2].

Capecitabine (Xeloda)

Capecitabine was approved by the FDA in September 2001 to be used in combination therapy with docetaxel (Taxotere) for treating patients whose metastatic breast cancer has progressed after treatment with an anthracycline (eg, doxorubicin) [4]. Capecitabine is also approved as single agent therapy for metastatic breast or colorectal cancer.

Capecitabine is the first oral drug that works through enzymatic activation of fluorouracil (5-FU). Once in the body, capecitabine is converted into 5-FU by the naturally produced enzyme thymidine phosphorylase (TP) [3]. 5-FU exerts its ability to kill cancer cells by preventing DNA synthesis.

The most common adverse events reported include diarrhea, nausea, vomiting, painful inflammation of the mouth, fatigue, painful swelling or redness of the hands or feet, and bone marrow suppression [4]. These side effects are reversible when treatment is stopped or the dose is reduced.

Docetaxel (Taxotere)

The FDA originally approved Docetaxel in 1996 for patients whose advanced breast cancer has progressed despite treatment with standard cancer treatments, such as doxorubicin. In November 2002, it was approved for first-line treatment in combination with cisplatin for treatment of unresectable, locally advanced, or metastatic non-small cell lung cancer (NSCLC) [2,4]. At the time docetaxel was approved, it became the only chemotherapy agent approved for newly diagnosed NSCLC patients and for those with recurrent disease [3].

Docetaxel works by inhibiting cancer cell division through essentially "freezing" the cell's internal skeleton, which is comprised of microtubules. Microtubules assemble and disassemble during a cell cycle. Docetaxel promotes their assembly and blocks their disassembly, thereby preventing cancer cells from dividing, resulting in cancer cell death [3].

The most common adverse events reported with docetaxel are neutropenia, anemia, nausea, vomiting, fluid retention, asthenia (ie, loss of strength), pain, and alopecia. Other side effects include diarrhea, weight loss, stomatitis, infection, hemoptysis, and constipation. Less common side effects include thrombocytopenia, hypersensitivity reactions, myalgia, arthralgia, and dehydration [2].

Innovations in biotherapy

Targeted therapy is another innovation in the treatment of cancer. Immunotherapy, or biotherapy, involves the use of the body's immune system to fight cancer. Targeted therapies are novel strategies in cancer treatment [5]. These therapies focus on cell signaling and other biologic ways that tumors grow and develop [6]. Targeted therapy involves the use of substances that can locate and bind to cancer cells. These substances block a specific cell pathway to prevent cells from dividing and metastasizing. Targeted therapies can usually spare normal cells from the side effects associated with conventional treatments for cancer [7]. Therapies using monoclonal antibodies in targeting cancer cells most likely account for most of the newest innovations in cancer treatment in the past few years.

Our immune system works by distinguishing self from non-self. When a foreign substance, or antigen, is detected by the body, antibodies attack that antigen. Each antibody has the capacity to recognize and bind to one antigen that is located on cell surfaces.

There are several types of biotherapy. One type, the monoclonal antibody (MAB), was developed decades ago through immunizing mice with an antigen. Today, human monoclonal antibodies and chimeric antibodies, which usually consist of human and mouse antibodies (70% and 30%, respectively), are used as part of the arsenal against cancer. Regardless of the source of the antibody, MABs are specific to a particular antigen. MABs are used to treat cancer because of their ability to recognize certain proteins that are present on the cell surfaces of cancer cells. The MAB then locks onto those proteins and triggers the immune system to attack cancer cells [8].

One method to enhance the efficacy of a MAB is to combine it with another form of cancer treatment, such as chemotherapy or radioactive substances. In this case, the monoclonal antibody will target and latch onto the cancer cell through a specific protein on the cancer cell surface, and then the cancer-killing therapy will cause death of the cancer cell [9].

Ibritumomab tiuxetan (Zevalin)

Ibritumomab tiuxetan is the first of two radiopharmaceuticals that were approved by the FDA. Radiopharmaceuticals are MABs with a radioactive source attached for cancer-killing effect. Ibritumomab tiuxetan was approved in April 2002 as part of the treatment for relapsed or refractory low-grade follicular or transformed B-cell non-Hodgkin's lymphoma [4].

Ibritumomab tiuxetan is used in combination with rituximab (Rituxan), another MAB. They target the CD20 protein on B-cells and then a high dose of radiation is delivered to the tumor. CD20 is a protein that is expressed on normal and most malignant B-cells. The therapy is a two-part procedure. First, the patient receives rituximab and a form of ibritumomab tiuxetan along with a low dose of a radioactive chemical, indium-111, for screening purposes. If the cancer cells are targeted appropriately, the patient receives a second dose of rituximab with a different radioactive chemical, yttrium 90, for actual cancer treatment. Stem cells are not affected with this therapy because they do not possess the CD20 protein [10].

Severe infusion reactions have been reported with this regimen and toxicities are more significant as compared with treatment involving rituximab alone. There is substantial occurrence of myelosuppression, life-threatening infection, and hemorrhage. Severe infusion reactions have also been reported, including hypoxia, pulmonary infiltrates, acute respiratory distress syndrome, myocardial infarction, ventricular fibrillation, and cardiogenic shock. For this reason, ibritumomab tiuxetan is only approved for patients who have failed other therapies [4,11].

Tositumomab and iodine 131 tositumomab (Bexxar)

Tositumomab and iodine 131 tositumomab is another radiopharmaceutical combination that was approved by the FDA. It was approved in June 2003 for the treatment of patients who have CD20 positive follicular non-Hodgkin's lymphoma that is untreatable with rituximab (another MAB), and have suffered relapse following chemotherapy [2]. The MAB, tositumomab, recognizes the CD20 on the lymphoma cells, locks onto the protein, and triggers the immune system to attack the cancer cells. Iodine 131, the radioactive substance attached to the MAB, delivers radiation directly to the cells with CD20 protein and kills the lymphoma B-cells. The lymphoma cells receive higher concentrations of radiation than normal cells, thereby minimizing toxicity [2].

The tositumomab and iodine 131 tositumomab combination is administered over 7 to 14 days. Treatments are traditionally administered a week apart, but may be given on the same day. Patients are usually hospitalized for the second treatment to minimize radiation exposure [2].

Adverse effects reported from tositumomab and iodine 131 tositumomab therapy include flu-like symptoms, allergic reaction (eg, bronchospasm, itchiness, rash), chills, weakness, nausea, and rhinitis. The most serious effects are related to pancytopenia and its sequela-like hemorrhage, and sepsis. Less common side effects include pneumonia, pleural effusion, and dehydration. Development of secondary leukemia has also been reported [2].

Alemtuzumab (Campath)

Alemtuzumab was the first MAB that was approved by the FDA for the treatment of chronic lymphocytic leukemia (CLL) [12]. The FDA approved it in August 2001 for treatment of B-cell CLL in patients who have been treated with alkylating agents and who have failed treatment with fludarabine [13].

Alemtuzumab binds to the CD52 protein that is present on the cell surfaces of malignant lymphocytes. After binding to the protein, it causes lysis and death of the cancer cells [5].

The most common adverse events reported from treatment with alemtuzumab include pancytopenia, fever and chills, sepsis, pneumonia, nausea, vomiting, rash, and hypotension [13]. Concern has also been expressed regarding infusion reactions and the development of opportunistic infections related to immunosuppression [12].

Imatinib mesylate (Gleevec)

The FDA approved imatinib mesylate in December 2003 as a second-line treatment for patients with Philadelphia chromosome-positive chronic myeloid leukemia (CML) following failure of treatment with interferon-alpha. This drug was approved for treating CML patients either in blast crisis, which is a phase of CML when there is a very high number of immature and abnormal white blood cells (WBCs) in the bone marrow and blood, in accelerated phase, or in chronic phase of the disease. It received accelerated approval for treatment of newly diagnosed CML in December 2002. Regular approval is still pending for this latter indication.

Protein kinases are enzymes that transfer phosphate from adenosine triphosphate (ATP) to specific amino acids on proteins. Transfer of phosphorus onto proteins causes activation of signal-transduction pathways,which results in cell growth. Several protein kinases are overexpressed in some types of cancer. There are two subfamilies of protein kinases, one of which is protein tyrosine kinase. One type of tyrosine kinase is Bcr-Abl, which is created by the Philadelphia chromosome and is therefore overexpressed in CML [14]. Bcr-Abl decreases the response to stimuli for apoptosis (ie, programmed cell death). CML is dependent on tyrosine kinase activity of Bcl-Abl [15].

Imatinib mesylate inhibits ATP binding sites of tyrosine kinase enzymes and inhibits the enzyme tyrosine kinase from sending out the signal that is responsible for the production of mature and immature WBCs [4,14]. The drug blocks proliferation and induces apoptosis in cancer cells with Bcr-Abl genes [16].

The most common reported adverse events include nausea, muscle cramps, fatigue, diarrhea, headache, arthralgia, periorbital edema, myalgia, fluid retention, hemorrhage, musculoskeletal pain, and rash [2,13,14]. Imatinib mesylate was once considered a promising superstar drug, but while the standard of care for CML is currently imatinib mesylate, this agent is not considered the miracle cure that many hoped it would be [17,18].

Bortezomib (Velcade)

Bortezomib was approved by the FDA in June 2003 for treatment of patients who have multiple myeloma (ie, cancer of the plasma cells, which are the WBCs that produce antibodies), received at least two prior therapies, and experienced disease progression since the last therapy [19].

Bortezomib is a new class of cancer treatment. It inhibits proteasomes from functioning normally. Proteasomes are enzyme complexes found in cells that play a role in the function of cancer and normal cells. Proteasome inhibition prevents growth and division of cancer cells, and decreases some growth stimulants for tumor cells. The disrupted protein may cause tumor cells to undergo apoptosis by inhibiting the proteasome [4].

Adverse events reported in preliminary studies include immunosuppression, anxiety, blurred or double vision, weakness, anorexia, fever, nausea, fatigue, headache, drowsiness, and peripheral neuropathy. Bortezomib can also cause dehydration and orthostasis due to vomiting or diarrhea.

Gemtuzumab ozogomicin (Mylotarg)

Gemtuzumab ozogomicin was approved by the FDA in May 2000 for the treatment of patients aged 60 or older who have CD33 positive acute myeloid leukemia (AML) that has relapsed for the first time and who are poor candidates for cytotoxic therapy [4]. The CD33 protein is seen in 90% of cases of AML. It is absent on normal stem cells. The MAB recognizes the CD33 protein on leukemic cell surfaces, targets the leukemic cells, and delivers a potent chemotherapy called calicheamycin. The calicheamycin exerts cancer-killing effects on the leukemic cells and leaves other cells healthy [20].

Adverse events include temporary bone marrow suppression, anemia, thrombocytopenia, infection, bleeding, stomatitis, liver problems, and rash. No major organ damage has been reported [4].

Angiogenesis inhibition

Biotherapy may also be used as an inhibitor of angiogenesis to combat cancer. Angiogenesis involves the formation and growth of new blood vessels, and is vital for cancer metastasis. If new blood vessels are unable to form, a tumor will not have an adequate blood supply. The tumor will be deprived of essential nutrients and therefore may either grow more slowly, cease cell growth, or shrink and die.

Arsenic trioxide (Trisenox)

The FDA approved arsenic trioxide in September 2000 for the treatment of patients with acute promyelocytic leukemia (APL) who have not responded to, or have relapsed following exposure to, the first-line therapy composed of all trans-retinoic acid and chemotherapy with anthracyclines [4]. Arsenic trioxide is now being evaluated for efficacy in treatment of CML and AML in patients who have not responded to other regimens.

The mechanism of action of arsenic trioxide is not completely understood. The drug evidently affects several intracellular signal transduction pathways and causes changes in cellular function. These actions may result in inhibition of angiogenesis and initiate apoptosis [21]. It is also suggested that arsenic trioxide causes damage to or degradation of the fusion protein PML-RAR alpha, which induces apoptosis and differentiation [4].

Adverse events that have been reported with arsenic trioxide administration include chills, decreased urine output, dysrhythmias, muscle pain, shortness of breath, loss of appetite, seizures, dry mouth, headache, weakness, nausea, vomiting, abdominal discomfort, skin changes, fluid accumulation, sore throat, cough, eye pain, increased thirst, mood changes, fatigue, and numbness of hands, feet and lips. Some patients also developed a prolongation of the QT interval, which can cause fatal arrhythmias [4].

Epidermal growth factor receptors

Epidermal growth factor receptor (EGFR) is present on non-malignant cells but is often overexpressed in cancer cells [22]. Growth factors and their receptors play an important role in the development and progression of cancer and they help cancer cells get repaired when they are damaged by traditional cancer treatments [23]. Given the enhanced understanding of cell biology, specifically cell signaling, therapies that target EGFR are novel strategies under investigation [24]. A number of ways are available to block the EGFR pathway. These include use of tyrosine kinase inhibitors and anti-EGFR MABs [25]. Studies with tyrosine kinase inhibitors are showing promise [22,26].

Tyrosine kinase is an enzyme within a cell. These enzymes attach a phosphate group to tyrosine, which is an amino acid. When phosphorus attaches, tyrosine kinase can trigger a series of events in a signaling system that stimulates cancer cell growth. Tyrosine kinase inhibitors block the ability of the protein tyrosine kinases to function. They bind to the enzyme instead of the phosphorus, causing rapid cell death [27].

Gefitinib (Iressa)

The FDA approved gefitinib in May 2003 for single-agent therapy of locally advanced or metastatic non-small cell lung cancer (NSCLC) that has progressed despite treatment with other chemotherapy, specifically platinum-based agents and docetaxel. Gefitinib is not recommended for use in combination with chemotherapy [2,3].

Gefitinib blocks EGFRs and tyrosine kinase activity [5,28]. Its mode of action is to block signals within cancer cells, thereby preventing these cells from growing and dividing. This is known as inhibition of signal transduction [8]. EGFR-tyrosine kinase plays an essential role in the growth, invasion, metastasis, and angiogenesis of NSCLC and its resistance to apoptosis [29,30].

The most common adverse events reported with gefitinib are rash and diarrhea. Data from clinical trials reveal mixed results in efficacy of treatment. Potential roles for this therapy are continuing to be investigated.

Bevacizumab (Avastin)

Bevacizumab is a monoclonal antibody that acts as an antiangiogenesis agent. It targets and blocks the protein vascular endothelial growth factor (VEGF), fitting like a lock and key into the receptor of a cell surface, and stopping VEGF from developing new blood vessels. It received FDA approval in February 2004 as a first-line treatment of patients with metastatic colorectal cancer. Bevacizumab was recently reported to be effective in the treatment of advanced colorectal cancer, demonstrating improvement in overall survival [31]. This agent is also being studied for efficacy in renal cell carcinoma, prostate cancer, and non-Hodgkin's lymphoma.

Common adverse events that have been reported in clinical trials include allergic reactions, fever, chills, mouth sores, constipation, nausea, vomiting, headache, fatigue, muscle aches, nose bleeds, hemoptysis, hematemesis, rash, thrombocytopenia, sore throat, pain, cough, shortness of breath, and neutropenia [2].

Cetuximab (Erbitux)

Cetuximab is an MAB that targets EGFR. It was approved in February 2004 for use either in combination with irinotecan or as a single-agent therapy in treating patients who have metastatic colorectal cancer. It remains under investigation for use in pancreatic, non-small cell lung, and head and neck cancers. Erb-1 is an EGFR that is stimulated by epidermal growth factor. Activation of EGFR causes a signaling cascade that leads to DNA synthesis, cell proliferation, differentiation, migration, and angiogenesis [5]. Cetuximab competes for the binding of EGFR and removes the receptor from the cell surface [5,43].

The adverse events reported in treatments involving cetuximab have been mild and include diarrhea, decreased WBCs, an acne-like rash, and vomiting. Some severe events were experienced in patients who received cetuximab as a single-agent therapy, including difficulty breathing, weakness, and pain [2].

Hormonal therapy

Many advances have been made with hormonal therapies in the fight against cancer. One example of this is the use of aromatase inhibitors (AIs), a newer class of hormone therapies [31].

Estrogen stimulates many types of breast cancers to grow. This group of breast cancers is categorized as estrogen-receptor positive (ER+). These cancerous cells have receptors that bind to estrogen hormones, facilitating tumor growth. The enzyme aromatase produces estrogen in addition to the ovaries. Aromatase is found in the liver and fatty tissues. AIs interfere with the body's use of aromatase, thereby decreasing the amount of estrogen produced; they do not affect the estrogen produced by the ovaries. When the amount of estrogen generated is reduced, there is less available for cancer cells to use for growth [32]. Currently there are three commercially available, FDA-approved AIs: anastrazole (Arimidex), exemestane (Aromasin), and letrozole (Femera). AIs work differently from tamoxifen, which blocks the ability of the tumor to use estrogen [2].

The FDA approved the use of AIs for postmenopausal women only, because the ovaries have stopped producing estrogen in these women. Despite menopause, the body continues to have low levels of estrogen circulating because the enzyme aromatase converts other hormones in the body into estrogen. AIs prevent conversion of these other hormones (ie, androgens) to estrogen, thereby decreasing the availability of the hormone needed for tumor growth [32].

Anastrazole (Arimidex)

The FDA approved anastrazole in September 2002 as adjuvant (ie, supplementary) treatment for postmenopausal women who have locally advanced or metastatic breast cancer [33]. Anastrazole was the first hormonal treatment approved for adjuvant therapy since tamoxifen.

Data from a study reported in December 2002 revealed that Arimedex was superior to tamoxifen in postmenopausal women with early ER+ breast cancer. Arimedex decreased the risk of breast cancer 17% more than tamoxifen alone and decreased the chance of breast cancer developing in the other breast by approximately 80% (60% better than tamoxifen) [32].

The reported adverse events are similar to those experienced in tamoxifen therapy. An increase in musculoskeletal incidents such as arthritis, arthralgia, hypercholesterolemia, and fractures of the spine, hip, and wrist, and a decrease in lumbar spine and total hip bone density, have been reported [2]. However, women have experienced fewer hot flashes and venous thrombotic and ischemic cerebrovascular events, and less vaginal bleeding, vaginal discharge, and occurrences of endometrial cancer than those receiving tamoxifen. Other adverse events include depression, stiffness, hair thinning, pharyngitis, weight gain, nausea, and vomiting.

Exemestane (Aromasin)

Exemestane is approved for postmenopausal women for whom tamoxifen has stopped working. Women who take tamoxifen to prevent recurrence following cancer treatment and develop advanced cancer during this time, or sometime afterwards, are candidates for this therapy [34].

Adverse events reported with the use of exemestane include fatigue, nausea, vomiting, hot flashes, pain, depression, insomnia, anxiety, shortness of breath, dizziness, headache, edema of arms and legs, abdominal pain, increased or loss of appetite, cough, flu-like symptoms, diarrhea, hypertension, weight gain, hair thinning, and constipation.

Letrozole (Femera)

The FDA initially approved letrozole in 1997 for women with breast cancer who did not respond to antiestrogen therapy [4]. Letrozole is now used with postmenopausal women who have locally advanced or metastatic breast cancer [34]. In January 2001 it was approved as a first-line therapy for postmenopausal women with metastatic breast cancer [4].

A lower incidence of adverse events has been reported in treatment with letrozole than with tamoxifen. Such events include pain, dyspnea, loss of appetite, vaginal dryness, muscle or joint pain, hot flashes, nausea, fatigue, night sweats, headache, and shortness of breath.

A recent study found that breast cancer survivors who took letrozole after completing 5 years of tamoxifen therapy were less likely to have disease recurrence than those who did not [35].

Fulvestrant (Faslodex)

The FDA approved fulvestrant in April 2002 for the treatment of hormone receptor-positive metastatic breast cancer in postmenopausal women with disease progression following antiestrogen therapy (eg, tamoxifen). Fulvestrant is an estrogen-receptor antagonist. While fulvestrant is a type of hormonal therapy, its mechanism of action is different from AIs, which reduce the amount of estrogen in a woman's body, and tamoxifen, which blocks the estrogen receptor in breast cancer cells. Fulvestrant instead targets and destroys the estrogen receptors in breast cancer cells, representing another method that can be used to treat ER+ breast cancer [3,13].

Reported adverse events with fulvestrant therapy include nausea, vomiting, constipation, diarrhea, abdominal pain, back pain, headache, hot flashes, and pharyngitis [2,13].

Leuprolide (Eligard)

Leuprolide was initially approved in January 2002 for treatment of prostate cancer. In July 2002, a sustained release product was approved, thereby changing the dosing frequency from every month to every 3 months. In February 2003, it was also approved for the palliative treatment of advanced prostate cancer [3].

Leuprolide is a luteinizing hormone-releasing hormone agonist. It decreases testosterone levels, thereby suppressing tumor growth in patients with hormone-responsive prostate cancer [3].

Reported adverse events associated with leuprolide treatment include hot flashes, diaphoresis, fatigue, gastroenteritis, malaise, and dizziness.

Abarelix (Plenaxis)

The FDA approved abarelix in November 2003 for the treatment of symptoms of advanced prostate cancer for which there are no other therapeutic options. Abarelix is a gonadotropin-releasing hormone antagonist. It lowers testosterone, the hormone needed for most prostate cancers to grow [4].

The life-threatening nature of the adverse events associated with abarelix is the rationale for the drug's strict indications for use. The reported reactions include anaphylaxis associated with hypotension and fainting, and loss of consciousness. Patients receiving abarelix should be monitored for at least 30 minutes following administration. Less serious side effects include hot flashes, sleep disturbances, pain, back pain, breast enlargement or pain, and constipation [4].

In the pipeline

Several pharmacologic agents in various phases of development are being investigated for cancer treatment. Results of angiogenesis inhibitor studies conducted in mice were released in the late 1990s, demonstrating the effects of blocking VEGF, a protein released by tumors to recruit blood vessels [36]. As a result of these studies, several angiogenesis inhibitors are currently being investigated in clinical trials. The following are a few examples of agents under evaluation.

Epratuzumab

Epratuzumab was granted orphan drug status in January 2003. Orphan drug status is granted by the FDA as an incentive for companies to develop and investigate treatments of rare diseases that occur in fewer than 200,000 patients annually in the United States. Epratuzumab is a humanized monoclonal antibody that targets CD22 proteins. It is being investigated for efficacy in non-Hodgkin's lymphoma [37].

Virulizin

Virulizin was granted orphan status by the FDA in February 2001, and fast track status in June 2002 for the treatment of pancreatic cancer that is refractory to conventional first-line therapy with gemcitabine. Virulizin is a distinctive type of biotherapy derived from cow bile. It recruits killer cells, monocytes, and macrophages to attack cancer cells [3].

Oblimersen sodium (Genasense)

Bcl-2 is a protein expressed on several types of cancer cells. It prevents apoptosis, increases the potential for metastasis, and promotes resistance to antineoplastic therapies, such as chemotherapy, radiation therapy, and MABs [38]. High levels of Bcl-2 block the release of cytochrome C from mitochondria, thereby preventing apoptosis [39].

Oblimersen sodium is a unique type of agent known as an antisense drug. It inhibits the production of the protein Bcl-2 and is administered before antineoplastic therapy to potentially enhance efficacy of treatment. Oblimersen sodium binds to part of the Bcl-2 mRNA sequence of cancer cells, resulting in cell degradation [40]. Oblimersen sodium is being evaluated for efficacy in combination with chemotherapy in patients with relapsed non-Hodgkin's lymphoma [41].

Advexin

Advexin was granted fast track status by the FDA in September 2003 for the treatment of patients with recurrent, unresectable squamous cell carcinoma of the head and neck [3]. Advexin supplies high concentrations of p53 in cancer tissue. p53 is a protein that has tumor suppressor effects on cells; it stops the cancer cell's signal to grow. The primary role of p53 is to recognize when a cell is damaged by mutation and initiate repair of the damaged cell by stopping cell growth. If the cell is damaged beyond repair, p53 activates the apoptosis pathway to prevent the cell from growing out of control [42].

Summary

Cancer is a complex group of diseases. Many of the current treatment modalities available provide limited effectiveness and significant side effects. This circumstance creates a challenge for health care providers. There is great need for the development of innovative therapies that increase efficacy and decrease morbidity [44].

In general, chemotherapeutic agents are unable to distinguish cancer cells from normal cells. As a result of therapy, patients may develop significant myelosuppression. Patients who are undergoing chemotherapy need to be observed for signs of hematologic and nonhematologic toxicities. Patients should be advised that periodic blood tests are indicated to monitor for anemia, neutropenia, and thrombocytopenia. If myelosuppression develops, measures to prevent complications such as bleeding and infection are indicated. Strategies to combat fatigue should also be discussed.

Understanding of the biology of cancer has increased significantly in recent years. As knowledge of the science grows, new therapies are developed and clinical trials are initiated to investigate feasibility and efficacy of agents. Many of these trials involve agents that target specific biologic processes of cancer.

While the complexities of cancer treatment are prolonging the life expectancy of patients who have the disease, patients are presenting with increasing numbers and types of morbidities. Nurses need to be aware of the rationale for treatment, mechanism of action of the agents administered, and expected toxicities of therapies. With this knowledge, symptoms can be identified earlier, life-threatening sequela can possibly be averted, and patients and families can be educated about what to expect and how to make knowledgeable decisions about treatment options. Enhancing patients' knowledge base may also increase their adherence to challenging therapies.

References

[1] Hochster HS. Opportunities for newer agents in combination with oxaliplatin. Semin Oncol 2003;30(4 Suppl 15):62–7.

[2] National Cancer Institute. Available at: http://www.cancer.gov. Accessed December, 2003.

[3] Doctor's Guide Channel. Available at http://www.docguide.com. Accessed November, 2003.

[4] Food and Drug Administration. Available at: http://www.fda.gov. Accessed December, 2003.

[5] Abou-Jawde R, Choueiri T, Alemany C, Mekhail T. An overview of targeted treatments in cancer. Clin Ther 2003;25(8):2121–37.

[6] Gridelli C, Rossi A, Maione P. Treatment of non-small-cell lung cancer: state of the art and development of new biologic agents. Oncogene 2003;22(42):6629–38.

[7] Gale DM. Molecular targets in cancer therapy. Semin Oncol Nurs 2003;19(3):193–205.

[8] Cancer BACUP. Available at: http://www.cancerbacup.org. Accessed December, 2003.

[9] Lymphoma Information Network. Available at: http://www.lymphomaininfo.net. Accessed December, 2003.

[10] National Cancer Institute. Available at: http://www.nci.nih.gov. Accessed December, 2003.

[11] American Pharmacists Association and National Association of Boards of Pharmacy. Available at: http://www.pharmacist.com. Accessed December, 2003.

[12] Mavromatis B, Chesen BD. Monoclonal antibody therapy for chronic lymphocytic leukemia. J Clin Oncol 2003;21(9):1874–81.

[13] Center Watch. Clinical Trials Listing Service. Available at: http://www.centerwatch.com. Accessed December, 2003.

[14] Lyseng-Williamson K, Jarvis B. Imatinib. Drugs 2001;61(12):1765–74.

[15] Savage DG, Antman KH. Drug therapy: imatinib mesylate-a new oral targeted therapy. N Engl J Med 2002;346(9):683–93.

[16] Druker BJ, Talpuz M, Resta DJ, Peng B, Buchdunger E, Ford JM, et al. Efficacy and safety of a specific inhibitor of the BCR-ABL tyrosine kinase in chronic myeloid leukemia. N Engl J Med 2001;19(3):193–205.

[17] Ault P, Kaled S, Rios MB. Management of molecular-targeted therapy for chronic myelogenous leukemia. J Am Acad Nurse Pract 2003;15(7):292–6.

[18] van Vlaanderen E. What happened to the "glee" in Gleevac? Clin Advis 2003;6(1):42–8.

[19] Multiple Myeloma Research Foundation. Available at: http://www.multiplemyeloma.org. Accessed December, 2003.

[20] Applebaum FR. Update on treatment for acute myeloid leukemia. Oncology Special Edition 2003;6:45–9.

[21] Miller WH, Schipper HM, Lee JS, Singer J, Waxman S. Mechanisms of action of arsenic trioxide. Cancer Res 2002;62(14):3893–903.

[22] Baselga J. Why the epidermal growth factor receptor? The rationale for cancer therapy. Oncologist 2002;7(Suppl 4):2–8.

[23] Spencer-Cisek PA. The role of growth factors in malignancy: a focus on the epidermal growth factor receptor. Semin Oncol Nurs 2002;18(2 Suppl 2):13–9.

[24] Sridhar SS, Seymour L, Shephard FA. Inhibitors of epidermal-growth-factor receptors: a review of clinical research with a focus on non-small-cell lung cancer. Lancet Oncol 2003; 4(7):397–406.

[25] Waxman ES, Herbst RS. The role of epidermal growth factor receptor in the treatment of colorectal carcinoma. Semin Oncol Nurs 2002;18(2 Suppl 2):20–9.

[26] Riddle J, Lee P, Purdom M. The epidermal growth factor receptor as a novel target for cancer therapy: case studies and clinical implications. Semin Oncol Nurs 2002;18(4 Suppl 4): 11–9.

[27] Parker Hughes Cancer Center. Available at: http://www.ih.org. Accessed December, 2003.

[28] Herbst RS, LoRusso PM, Purdom M, Ward D. Dermatologic side effects associated with gefitinib therapy: clinical experience and management. Clin Lung Cancer 2003;4(6):366–9.

[29] Herbst R, Langer C. Epidermal growth factor receptors as a target for cancer treatment: the emerging role of IMC-C225 in the treatment of lung and head and neck cancers. Semin Oncol(1 Supp 4):27–36.

[30] Ciardiello F, Tortora G. A novel approach in the treatment of cancer: targeting the epidermal growth factor receptor. Clin Cancer Res 2001;7:2958–70.

[31] Caley BA, Reidenbach F. Expanding options for advanced breast cancer. Cure 2003;2(3): 47–54.

[32] Breastcancer.org. Available at: http://www.breastcancer.org. Accessed December, 2003.

[33] Buzdar A. Anastrozole as adjuvant therapy for early-stage breast cancer: implications of the ATAC trial. Clin Breast Cancer 2003;4(Suppl 1):S42–8.

[34] National Alliance of Breast Cancer Organizations. Available at: http://www.nabco.org. Accessed December, 2003.

[35] Bryant J, Wolmark N. Letrozole after tamoxifen for breast cancer—what is the price of success? N Engl J Med 2003;349(19):1855–7.

[36] War On Cancer. Available at: http://www.witts.org. Accessed November, 2003.

[37] Juweid M. Technology evaluation: epratuzumab, immunogenics/amgen. Curr Opin Mol Ther 2003;5(2):192–8.

[38] Klasa RJ, Gillum AM, Klem RE, Frankel SR. Oblimersen bcl-2 antisense: facilitating apoptosis in anticancer treatment. Antisense Nucleic Acid Drug Dev 2002;12(3):193–213.

[39] Multiple Myeloma Research Foundation. Available at: http://www.multiplemyeloma.org. Accessed December, 2003.

[40] Jansen B, Zangemeister-Wittke U. Antisense therapy for cancer—the time of truth. Lancet Oncol 2002;3(11):672–83.

[41] Waters JS, Webb A, Cunningham D, Clarke PA, Raynaud F, di Stefano F, et al. Phase I clinical and pharmacokinetic study of bcl-2 antisense oligonucleotide therapy in patients with non-Hodgkin's lymphoma. J Clin Oncol 2000;18:1812–23.

[42] PSL Group. Available at: http://www.pslgroup.com. Accessed December, 2003.

[43] Waksal HW. Role of an anti-epidermal growth factor receptor in treating cancer. J Clin Oncol 2002;20:719–26.

[44] Stull DM. Targeted therapies for the treatment of leukemia. Semin Oncol Nurs 2003;19(2): 90–7.

ELSEVIER
SAUNDERS

Nurs Clin N Am 40 (2005) 95–105

NURSING
CLINICS
OF NORTH AMERICA

New Developments in Antidepressant Therapy

Karen S. Ward, PhD, RN, COI

School of Nursing, Box 81, Middle Tennessee State University,
Murfreesboro, TN 37132, USA

Treating depression is a challenging task for clinicians. Even with an increasing arsenal of psychotherapeutic medications, this client population tends to be demanding and energy-depleting. To help nursing students identify who among their clients are depressed, they are taught the strategy of asking themselves how they feel after prolonged interaction with the individual; if the student feels depressed, the client is probably depressed. Family members face this same emotional drain. Of course, the clients themselves are experiencing the most impact. Understanding and recognizing the symptoms of depression and being knowledgeable of the treatment intervention choices are critical elements in caring for depressed individuals and their families [1].

Clinical depression is not simply "the blues." Although what the general public usually refers to as "being depressed" is an undesirable condition, it does not typically refer to the life-threatening affliction of major depression. Individuals who truly suffer from depression cannot just "get over it" any more than a diabetic or someone with a broken leg can. Depression is considered a fatality risk. Over 90% of suicides occur when mental illness is present and, although not all of the incidents reflect a diagnosis of depression, most have a depressive component [2]. The World Health Organization cites depression as the leading cause of life-long disability [3]. Many researchers are urging health care providers to address this serious health problem more aggressively [4–6].

To date, there have been no conclusive research findings that identify the exact etiology of depression. Different theories provide ways of explaining the condition, falling under three main categories: (1) psychological factors, (2) biochemical factors, and (3) evolutionary factors [1]. Most likely, a variety of factors convene to cause the symptoms of major depression.

E-mail address: kward@mtsu.edu

0029-6465/05/$ - see front matter © 2005 Elsevier Inc. All rights reserved.
doi:10.1016/j.cnur.2004.08.008   ***nursing.theclinics.com***

Clients with major depression experience feelings of deep sadness, helplessness, and hopelessness. They see no way out of their situation and often feel guilty over the fact that they are so depressed, creating a vicious cycle of worsening depression and symptomatology, possibly culminating in a suicide attempt.

Depression is compounded by sleep disturbances and eating problems (eg, overeating, loss of appetite). As clients continue to withdraw from family and friends, they become even less interested in life around them. Their day-to-day tasks become difficult as a result of loss of energy and the inability to concentrate. Diminished productivity is one of the significant manifestations of the illness, as seen in Box 1 [1,4].

A short history

Treating mental health problems with medications is a relatively new intervention. Interest in chemicals that might affect mental disorders really developed in 1952, when it was discovered that chlorpromazine (Thorazine) reduced the hallucinations of psychotic patients and allowed them to remain calm for limited periods [1]. For many years, it was difficult to connect the right person with the right dosage of the right drug. When a new drug was discovered it tended to be prescribed for all psychiatric clients regardless of their symptoms. Sometimes, if a treatment didn't work for everyone, it was set aside as noneffective. As research has expanded the knowledge of brain functioning and chemical action, greater specificity is possible. Researchers are now exploring which chemical combinations target behaviors symptomatic of each psychiatric diagnostic category. Today, when medications are prescribed for clients with mental disturbances, there is much greater potential for symptom relief and better understanding of what to expect

---

Box 1. Symptoms of major depression

D Depressed Mood
E Excitement gone
P Problems at work
R Risk for suicide
E Eating changes
S Sleep pattern disturbance
S Social withdrawal
I Irritability
O Overwhelming guilt
N No energy

with the drug. For this reason there is more hope than ever for symptom relief for all psychiatric clients, including those with depression.

Categories of interventions

There are several treatment modalities for individuals experiencing depression. Four main categories will be discussed briefly. Talking therapy, or psychotherapy, proves useful for most clients. Electroconvulsive therapy (ECT) was first tried on psychiatric clients when there was little else to choose from, and has made a comeback because it does seem to work with some clients. Bright light therapy has gained favor as a treatment of choice for certain depressed clients. Finally, increasing numbers of effective medications are available for use in reducing depressive symptoms.

Psychotherapy

Talking about problems has been shown to be helpful in many situations. However, since the advent of effective medication, it is common for individuals to ignore the value of counseling and interaction therapies [6,7]. Chronic disease of any kind puts stress on the individual. The assistance of a therapist, counselor, or support group is useful in discussing all aspects of the disease. From frustrations with relapse to concerns about medication side effects, sharing the experience with someone else can be a healing factor. There are several varieties of counseling, and clients may need to try a few before finding one that works for them. Clients and their families can benefit from psychotherapy whether or not the client's symptoms are the result of a chemical imbalance and can be treated with medication [1].

Electroconvulsive therapy

Cerletti and Beni first introduced electroconvulsive therapy (ECT) in the treatment of psychiatric clients in 1934. It involves placing electrodes on the client's head and passing an electrical current through the brain, thus inducing a seizure. Even today, it is unclear why ECT works for some people. Although ECT became unpopular, primarily because of its portrayal in films such as *One Flew Over the Cuckoo's Nest*, its usefulness in some cases is well-documented. Of the 15% of depressed clients who do not respond to pharmacotherapy, 90% are helped with ECT [1]. Significant differences exist today in the administration of ECT from the early days of its use. Among other changes, the actual electric current is at a lower voltage and the recipient receives a variety of medications to control the induced seizure, making the situation much safer than in the past. It has actually become the treatment of choice for clients who do not receive benefit from other treatment modalities or who are unable to take medication, such as pregnant women [1,7].

Bright light therapy

Although it is unclear why sitting under bright light for about 30 minutes each day may help alleviate depression, there are many people who can testify to its usefulness. It is thought that the light stimulates production of serotonin, but the exact mechanism is not known. Some feel that use of light in the morning helps to re-establish regular circadian rhythms. This therapy seems to produce no harmful results, because the light does not have to contain the full spectrum and therefore does not subject the client to unsafe rays. Similar treatment includes the use of rose or blue-green tinted glasses or light visors if clients do not respond to the "bright light" [1,7,8].

Pharmaceutical therapy

There are numerous medications on the market for treatment of depression. These antidepressants and other drugs vary both structurally and in their effectiveness with individual clients. Unfortunately, there is no sure way to identify which medication is best for any given client. However, it is reassuring to know that most clients receive some relief from their depression if the right medication is found [9,10].

With so many medications to choose from, research must be scrutinized to determine the quality of each study. Anderson [11] reviewed significant literature for issues that could guide practitioners in their own reading. He advocates the conduct of large randomized controlled trials and careful monitoring for bias in either sample selection or reporting. While not recommending any particular medications, he defines several areas to investigate when determining the best course of treatment. Issues facing the practitioner, such as deciding when to increase the dosage, when to switch medications, and when to discontinue drug use, are explored as problems because of the very individualized nature of medication response.

Another interesting issue has to do with the interaction of pharmaceutical sales representatives and nurses. Although physicians are accustomed to dealing with these sales representatives, Hemingway [12] points out that mental health nurse practitioners must now become proactive in learning to judge the information provided by pharmaceutical companies. Because nurses are now prescribing medications, they must evaluate the objectivity of any research presented.

Additional studies caution that financial sponsorship of research can have a significant effect on the results of a study and that the methodology in clinical trials should be carefully evaluated [13,14]. Bias on the part of the researcher can serve to devalue the research. Unfortunately, it is sometimes hard to discern bias if it is not expected. A major dilemma comes from the fact that the research is needed and the ones most interested in conducting it are the ones most likely to have the bias. This knowledge requires thoughtful review on the part of each practitioner.

Current medications

There are five main classes of antidepressant medications. These include monoamine oxidase inhibitors (MAOIs), cyclics, selective serotonin reuptake inhibitors (SSRIs), other antidepressants, and over the counter (OTC) or herbal remedies. Clearly, newer drugs are being developed and appear on the market every year, so it is doubtful that the final category of medication has been made available given the rapid explosion of knowledge about brain functioning and psychopathology. As previous research has shown, no one medication is going to work for everyone.

Monoamine oxidase inhibitors

The first drug used for treatment of depression was iproniazid, an antituberculosis agent. The serendipitous discovery was made that clients who were taking their tuberculosis medication regularly appeared happier. Structurally, iproniazid is an MAOI [1,10]. Depressed individuals exhibit lowered levels of monoamines (eg, serotonin, norepinephrine, and dopamine). By taking a medication that causes these neurotransmitters to accumulate, depression is eased (Table 1). However, as a result of the inhibition of monoamine oxidase, which is the enzyme that destroys excess neurotransmitters, another substance called tyramine also builds up. This buildup can cause an extreme rise in blood pressure, one that can even be fatal, especially if foods rich in tyramine are consumed. Because of significant problems with food and drug interactions, MAOIs are not the first choice for treatment, but because they do provide relief for certain patients who do not respond well to any of the other classes of medications, they remain on the market [1,10].

Cyclic antidepressants

Cyclic antidepressants were the first group of drugs to come onto the scene specifically for the treatment of depression (Table 2). Beginning in 1958, when imipramine (Tofranil) was introduced, cyclic antidepressants

Table 1
Representative monoamine oxidase inhibitors and their dosages

Specific monoamine oxidase inhibitor	Normal starting dose	Maintenance dose
Phenelzine (Nardil)	15 mg/d	15–60 mg/d
Tranylcypromine (Parnate)	10–30 mg/d	10–40 mg/d

Data from Fortinash KM, Worret PAH. Psychiatric mental health nursing. 3rd edition. St. Louis: Mosby; 2004; and Turkington C, Kaplan EF. Making the antidepressant decision. Chicago: Contemporary Books; 2001.

Table 2
Representative cyclic antidepressants and their dosages

Specific cyclic	Normal starting dose	Maintenance dose
Amitriptyline (Elavil, Endep)	25–50 mg/d	100–300 mg/d
Amoxapine (Asendin)	50 mg/d	100–400 mg/d
Clomipramine (Anafranil)	25 mg/d	100–250 mg/d
Desipramine (Norpramin)	25–50 mg/d	100–300 mg/d
Doxepin (Adapin, Sinequan)	25–50 mg/d	75–300 mg/d
Imipramine (Janimine, Tofranil)	25–50 mg/d	100–300 mg/d
Maprotiline (Ludiomil)	50 mg/d	75–225 mg/d
Nortriptyline (Pamelor, Aventyl)	25–50 mg/d	50–300 mg/d
Protriptyline (Vivactil)	10 mg/d	15–60 mg/d
Trimipramine (Surmontil)	25–50 mg/d	75–300 mg/d

Data from Fortinash KM, Worret PAH. Psychiatric mental health nursing. 3rd edition. St. Louis: Mosby; 2004; and Turkington C, Kaplan EF. Making the antidepressant decision. Chicago: Contemporary Books; 2001.

remained the drugs of choice until the SSRIs were developed. The cyclic medications work by increasing the norepinephrine and serotonin levels in the brain, rather than acting as central nervous system stimulants or monoamine oxidase inhibitors. The side effects are the main drawback to the cyclic antidepressants; dry mouth, blurred vision and other anticholinergic reactions, sedation, cardiotoxicity, and risk of overdose commonly occur with administration of these medications. Many people find that the benefits do not outweigh the bothersome side effects. However, for some clients experiencing depression, the cyclics are the drugs of choice [1,10].

Selective serotonin reuptake inhibitors

Selective serotonin reuptake inhibitors (SSRIs) are widely used drugs for the treatment of depression (Table 3). The first SSRI, fluxetine (Prozac), was

Table 3
Representative selective serotonin reuptake inhibitors and their dosages

Specific selective serotonin reuptake inhibitor	Normal starting dose	Maintenance dose
Citalopram (Celexa)	20 mg/d	20–40 mg/d
Escitalopram oxalate (Lexapro)	10 mg/d	10–20 mg/d
Fluvoxamine (Luvox)	50 mg/d	100–300 mg/d
Fluxetine (Prozac)	5–20 mg/d	20–80 mg/d
Paroxetine (Paxil)	10–20 mg/d	20–50 mg/d
Sertraline (Zoloft)	50–100 mg/d	50–200 mg/d

Data from Fortinash KM, Worret PAH. Psychiatric mental health nursing. 3rd edition. St. Louis: Mosby; 2004; and Sternbeck H. Serotonin syndrome: how to avoid, identify, & treat dangerous drug interactions. Current Psychiatry Online [serial online]. May 2003;2(5). Available at: http://www.currentpsychiatry.com/2003_05/0503_serotonin.asp.

introduced in 1988 and several other versions have followed. Their inhibition is at the point of 5-hydroxy-tryptamine (5-HT) reuptake, causing an increase of that substance in the synapse of nerve fibers. It is anticipated that additional SSRIs will be put on the market as research progresses. This class of drugs offers the advantage of being effective in controlling depression whileand causing far fewer side effects than their predecessors. Each of the drugs in this class produces different side effects, which can sometimes be helpful in determining which one to select for a given client.

Of most concern in administering these medications is the possibility of serotonin syndrome, which can result from interaction with other drugs, including MAOIs. This syndrome can be life-threatening and requires hospitalization. It is similar to neuroleptic malignant syndrome, which occurs with the antipsychotic medications. Symptoms include euphoria, drowsiness, sustained rapid eye movement, restlessness, muscle twitching, rigidity, high body temperature, shivering, diarrhea, mental status changes, and loss of consciousness [15].

For most people suffering from depression, the SSRIs are the drugs of choice, but they do not work for everyone; it is not possible to predict which client will benefit from any particular medication. However, as a result of their widespread and reasonably successful treatment, they are often the first drugs prescribed [1,10,16].

Other antidepressants

The final group of medications prescribed for depression includes five drugs that are not related to each other or to the other groups in their chemical composition (Table 4). They have all shown great promise in efficacy for treating depressed patients. Their discoveries have occurred when scientists experimented with the chemistry of pre-existing antidepressants, creating unique compounds. New drugs are developed regularly that become available for individuals with depression once FDA approval is granted. Because each of these antidepressants is unique, less information is

Table 4
Representative other antidepressants and their dosages

Specific antidepressant	Normal starting dose	Maintenance dose
Bupropion (Wellbutrin)	200 mg/d	300–450 mg/d
Mirtazapine (Remeron)	15 mg/d	15–45 mg/d
Nefazodone (Serzone)	200 mg/d	300–600 mg/d
Trazodone (Desyrel)	50 mg/d	150–500 mg/d
Venlafaxine (Effexor)	75 mg/d	150–350 mg/d

Data from Fortinash KM, Worret PAH. Psychiatric mental health nursing. 3rd edition. St. Louis: Mosby; 2004; and Turkington C, Kaplan EF. Making the antidepressant decision. Chicago: Contemporary Books; 2001.

available, and therefore an SSRI will most often be ordered first [10]. However, all of these medications have worked well with clients who were unable to obtain relief from other treatments.

Over-the-counter and herbal remedies

Various forms of natural remedies have been touted as treatment for all sorts of disorders. Although they can be purchased over the counter (OTC) and do not require a prescription, many still deserve serious consideration before they are taken. It has been difficult to establish whether or not these preparations provide any real help with depression or any other pathology, because (1) not as many clinical trials are available to provide convincing data, (2) the preparations themselves can vary in strength and purity, and (3) the health care community discourages many clients from using them in conjunction with, or in place of, their prescribed medications.

Despite the lack of data, herbal supplements need to be treated like any other medication. They may provide effective treatment, but they may also cause harmful side effects. Eventually, as more people become interested in these substances and report their pharmaceutical actions, and as more clinical trials are completed, data will be collected in sufficient quantities to predict outcomes. In the meantime, "may the buyer beware."

There are a few herbal substances that have specifically been promoted for use as antidepressant therapy. St. John's wort comes from the plant *Hypericum anagalloides* and is the most studied of all the medicinal plants. Research results have been mixed, but many claim that St. John's wort can work as an antidepressant for some people, particularly if the depression is mild. St. John's wort does produce side effects, but these are minor and seem to disappear with continued use. Because of adverse interactions when combined with MAOIs and SSRIs, St. John's wort should never be taken in combination with any of these traditional medications [1,7,10,17]. Despite its popularity, scientific research does not support the conviction that it is useful in the treatment of major depression [18].

Sam-e is another highly publicized OTC remedy. Brown and colleagues [6] think so highly of its ability to help those with depression that a complete plan for self-treatment is presented in a recent book. Sam-e is a naturally occurring substance produced by animals. There are a few studies that suggest Sam-e can be an effective antidepressant, but many questions remain. Interestingly, while it is available OTC in the United States, it is sold as a prescription drug in Europe [6,7,10].

A few additional substances have been promoted as effective antidepressants. *Ginkgo biloba* can be helpful to some people, particularly those over 50, as a mood-elevating substance. Valerian root is not used as an antidepressant, but because of its anti-anxiety effects, it may be helpful in treating insomnia. The same is true for kava extract [7]. The root of *rauwolfia* contains reserpine and other alkaloids and can cause depression, but ironically, in combination with certain cyclic antidepressants, some clients who have resistive depression have experienced positive results [17].

Patient considerations

Education is a key factor in helping individuals experience the greatest relief from their depression. Information on side effects should be provided to all clients and their families. Often the side effects will subside once the body has adjusted to the medication. If clients know this up front, they are more likely to persevere and continue treatment.

Clients should also be fully informed of any contraindications to taking antidepressant medication. They need to be aware of possible reasons why they cannot take certain drugs. Sharing their medical history with their health care provider is important in determining appropriateness of treatment.

Clients should also be told that stopping their medication abruptly can be detrimental. Although antidepressants are not addictive, there is evidence of a discontinuation syndrome when clients who use these medications on a long-term basis suddenly stop. The medications should be gradually reduced and then stopped to avoid this uncolmfortable situation [1,19].

The cost of these medications is significant. Clients who lack insurance need to be informed of financial assistance opportunities. Even with insurance, some individuals are responsible for such high copays or deductibles that they require assistance in paying for the drug. Referring patients to Web sites such as www.neddymeds.com and encouraging them to compare costs can be helpful. Because individuals suffering from depression often lack energy and the ability to concentrate, assistance with basic budgeting can be extremely helpful. It is important to keep in mind that there are hidden costs of depression. This group of clients not only incurs the actual medical costs, but also may suffer lost wages, general loss of potential, and significant loss of self-esteem and confidence when presented with future opportunities. Depression can be quite a burden—financially and otherwise [20–22].

The good news and the bad news

Clearly there is a great deal of good news for individuals suffering with depression. There is a large number of medications currently available and more entering the market all the time. Reboxetine (Vestra) and duloxetine HCl (Cymbalta) are new agents in the final stages of approval [10,23]. Some of the atypical antipsychotics such as aripiprazole (Abilify), clozapine (Clozoril), olanzapine (Zyprexa), and risperidone (Risperdal) are showing promise as treatment for depression, especially for those clients exhibiting depression along with other psychotic symptoms [24].

Employment of antidepressants in the treatment of other disorders is under investigation. Irritable bowel syndrome, hot flashes, generalized anxiety disorder, posttraumatic stress disorder, and premenstrual dysphoric syndrome are among those conditions currently being treated with antidepressants [25–28]. It is encouraging that medications continue to provide surprises concerning their usefulness.

The bad news is that there is still no reliable way to determine which medication will work best for each client. In many cases, research has not yet shown the exact mechanisms of action even for medications that do seem to work. Certain individuals receive no relief from their depressive symptoms despite trials of multiple antidepressants. Some individuals conclude that suicide is the only way out of their despair, others simply continue to suffer day after day.

Overall, however, there is hope. As new drugs emerge and become fully tested, research findings will pave the way for more medications to be developed. As more individuals discover effective treatments, human suffering and lifelong disability will decrease. Continuous new developments in antidepressant therapy will give many individuals the opportunity to live more fulfilling lives, free of despair and full of optimism.

References

[1] Fortinash KM, Worret PAH. Psychiatric mental health nursing. 3rd edition. St Louis: Mosby; 2004.
[2] Institute of Medicine. Reducing suicide: a national imperative. Washington, DC: National Academies Press; 2002.
[3] World Health Organization. World Health Report 2001. Mental health: new understanding, new hope. Geneva (Switzerland): World Health Organization; 2001.
[4] Insel TR, Charney DS. Research on major depression: strategies and priorities. JAMA 2003; 289:3167–8.
[5] Glass RM. Awareness about depression: important for all physicians. JAMA 2003;289: 3169–70.
[6] Brown R, Bottiglieri T, Colman C. Stop depression now. New York: GP Putnam's Sons; 1999.
[7] Quinn BP. The depression sourcebook. Los Angeles: Lowell House; 1997.
[8] Torpy JM, Lynm C, Glass RM. Depression. JAMA 2003;289:3198.
[9] Geddes JR, Carney SM, Davies C, et al. Relapse prevention with antidepressant drug treatment in depressive disorders: a systematic review. Lancet 2003;361:653–61.
[10] Turkington C, Kaplan EF. Making the antidepressant decision. Chicago: Contemporary Books; 2001.
[11] Anderson IM. Drug treatment of depression: reflections of the evidence. Ad in Psy Tr 2003;9: 11–20.
[12] Hemingway S. Mental health nursing and the pharmaceutical industry. Mental Health Practice 2003;7:22–3.
[13] Baker CB, Johnsrud MT, Crismon ML, Rosenheck RA, Woods SW. Quantitative analysis of sponsorship bias in economic studies of antidepressants. Br J Psychiatry 2003;183: 498–506.

[14] Stolk P, Ten Berg MJ, Hemels ME, Einarson TR. Meta-analysis of placebo rates in major depressive disorder trials. Ann Pharmacother 2003;37:1891–9.

[15] Sternbeck H. Serotonin syndrome: how to avoid, identify, & treat dangerous drug interactions. Current Psychiatry Online [serial online]. May 2003;2(5). Available at: http://www.currentpsychiatry.com. Accessed January 8, 2004.

[16] Forest Pharmaceuticals, Inc. How to measure your patients' depression. St. Louis (MO): Forest Pharmaceuticals, Inc.; 2003.

[17] Williamson EM. Drug interactions between herbal and prescription medicines. Drug Saf 2003;26:1075–92.

[18] Shelton R, Keller M, Gelenberg A, Dunner D, Hirschfeld R, Thase M, et al. Effectiveness of St John's wort in major depression: a randomized controlled trial. JAMA 2001;285:1978–86.

[19] Antai-Otong D. Antidepressant discontinuation syndrome. Perspect Psychiatr Care 2003; 39:127–9.

[20] Thomas CM, Morris S. Cost of depression among adults in England. Br J Psychiatry 2003; 183:498–506.

[21] Dewa CS, Hoch JS, Lin E, Patterson M, Goering P. Pattern of antidepressant use and duration of depression-related absence from work. Br J Psychiatry 2003;183:507–13.

[22] Knapp M. Hidden costs of mental illness. Br J Psychiatry 2003;183:477–8.

[23] Bailey KP. Physical symptoms comorbid with depression and the new antidepressant Duloxetine. J Psychosoc Nurs Ment Health Serv 2003;41(12):13–8.

[24] Bailey KP. Do atypical antipsychotic agents have a role in the treatment of depression? J Psychosoc Nurs Ment Health Serv 2003;41(10):12–6.

[25] Clouse RE. Antidepressants for irritable bowel syndrome. Gut 2003;52:598–9.

[26] Kaiser Permanente. Menopause: some women turn to antidepressants to quell hot flashes. Drug Week. January 23, 2004:319.

[27] Flynn CA, Chen YC. Antidepressants for generalized anxiety disorder. Am Fam Physician 2003;68:1757–8.

[28] Bisson JI, Kitchiner NJ. Early psychosocial and pharmacological interventions after traumatic events. J Psychosoc Nurs Ment Health Serv 2003;41:42–51.

ELSEVIER
SAUNDERS

NURSING
CLINICS
OF NORTH AMERICA

Nurs Clin N Am 40 (2005) 107–117

Multidimensional Pharmacologic Strategies for Diabetes

Ken W. Edmisson, ND, EdD, RNC, FNP

School of Nursing, Middle Tennessee State University, Box 81,
Murfreesboro, TN 37132, USA

The burden of adult diabetes in the United States has increased substantially over the last decade. Diabetes represents a serious health risk to millions of Americans. Diabetes among adults increased rapidly during the 1990s across all demographic groups and nearly all states. Researchers at the Centers for Disease Control and Prevention (CDC) found that the prevalence of diagnosed diabetes increased by 33% during this time [1].

Between 1990 and 1998, researchers at the CDC reported a 70% increase in diabetes among individuals aged 30 to 39, followed by an increase of 40% among those aged 40 to 49, and a 31% increase among those aged 50 to 59. Obesity has increased rapidly in the United States. The incidence of diabetes is highly correlated with the prevalence of obesity ($P < 0.001$) [1].

Approximately 800,000 new cases of diabetes are diagnosed each year. In 1998, over 16 million Americans suffered from diabetes. It is the seventh leading cause of death in this country and a major contributing factor to health problems such as heart disease, hypertension, renal disease, stroke, blindness, wound healing, and amputations [1]. Diabetes is the most common cause of end-stage renal disease in the United States, and hypertension contributes to cardiovascular morbidity and mortality in people who have diabetes. Hypertension and diabetes are particularly prevalent in certain populations, such as African Americans and Native Americans [2].

Traditional management strategies have included lifestyle modification, glucose control, and pharmacologic therapy. These management strategies were acceptable at one time, but more modern approaches have emerged that prove to be superior. These approaches place more emphasis on client education regarding lifestyle management, better glucose control, and

E-mail address: edmisson@mtsu.edu

0029-6465/05/$ - see front matter © 2005 Elsevier Inc. All rights reserved.
doi:10.1016/j.cnur.2004.08.009   *nursing.theclinics.com*

pharmacologic therapies that not only focus on glucose control but also target cholesterol and blood pressure levels.

Lifestyle effects and modification

Lifestyle modification is and has always been the first-line treatment of choice for diabetes management. Control of weight and glucose levels through diet and exercise is the first topic discussed with patients who have been newly diagnosed with diabetes after the disease has been explained. Exercise and proper diet are particularly beneficial to type 2 diabetics. Weight loss affords the body the ability to concentrate the insulin receptors, thereby enabling them to become more efficient in insulin sensitivity. Weight loss should be approached carefully; proper physical evaluation of the client is warranted before implementing an exercise regimen. Referral to an exercise specialist is also encouraged for those individuals who are not accustomed to routine physical exercise. The American Heart Association (AHA) and the American Diabetes Association (ADA) recommend 30 minutes of daily physical activity [3–5]. Box 1 provides examples of exercise that can be tolerated by diabetic patients who suffer loss of protective sensation (ie, neuropathies).

Weight loss is also achieved through dietary control. Dietary control is best achieved when there is a thorough understanding of proper nutrition and its effect on the body. A low-fat diet consisting of moderate sodium

---

Box 1. Exercises for diabetic patients with loss of protective sensation

Contraindicated exercise
Treadmill
Prolonged walking
Jogging
Step exercises

Recommended Exercise
Swimming
Bicycling
Rowing
Chair exercises
Arm exercises
Other non–weight-bearing exercises

From [23]. American Diabetes Association. Physical activity/exercise and diabetes. Diabetes Care 2004:27(suppl 1);S58–62; with permission.

intake and 160 to 300 g of carbohydrates per day is recommended [6]. Referral to a dietitian or nutritionist is also recommended. Box 2 provides goals for medical nutrition therapy that apply to all individuals who have diabetes.

Another lifestyle modification people who have diabetes must contend with is the need for continuous glucose monitoring and control. Proper instruction concerning the importance of glucose monitoring and how it is performed is essential. Client activity level and glucose fragility should be taken into consideration when determining the frequency of glucose monitoring.

The ADA "Standards of Medical Care for Patients with Diabetes Mellitus" recommends the fasting plasma glucose test for the screening and diagnosing of diabetes. Preprandial plasma glucose values of 90 to 130 mg/dL and peak postprandial levels below 180 mg/dL are recommended to maintain glucose control in the adult patient who has diabetes. A glycosylated hemoglobin (A1C) value below 7% is also recommended. An A1C should be obtained two times a year for individuals who maintain good glycemic control, or quarterly for patients who are not at goal or who have changed their therapy [3]. Table 1 illustrates A1C levels and their relationship to average plasma glucose levels between A1C assessments.

Box 2. Goals of medical nutrition therapy for diabetes

1. Attain and maintain optimal metabolic outcomes including:
   (a) Blood glucose levels in the normal range or as close to normal as is safely possible to prevent or reduce the risk for complications of diabetes;
   (b) A lipid and lipoprotein profile that reduces the risk for macrovascular disease;
   (c) Blood pressure levels that reduce the risk for vascular disease.
2. Modify nutrient intake and lifestyle as appropriate for the prevention and treatment of obesity, dyslipidemia, cardiovascular disease, hypertension, and nephropathy.
3. Improve health through healthy food choices and physical activity.
4. Address individual nutritional needs, taking into consideration personal and cultural preferences and lifestyle while respecting the individual's wishes and willingness to change.

From American Diabetes Association. Nutrition principles and recommendations in diabetes. Diabetes Care 2004:7(suppl 1);S36–46; with permission.

Table 1
Correlation between glycosylated hemoglobin (A1C) and mean plasma glucose levels

Hemoglobin	Mean plasma glucose	
A1C (%)	mg/dL	mmol/L
6	135	7.5
7	170	9.5
8	205	11.5
9	240	13.5
10	275	15.5
11	310	17.5
12	345	19.5

From [24]. American Diabetes Association Standards of medical care in diabetes. Diabetes Care 2004;27(Suppl 1):S15–35; with permission.

An annual influenza vaccine is recommended for all diabetic patients 6 months of age or older. At least one lifetime pneumococcal vaccination for adults with diabetes, as is a one-time revaccination for all previously immunized individuals under 64 years of age [3].

As with any management strategy, it is imperative that the primary care provider be involved. The provider must share in the responsibility of weight control and diet therapy, although glucose monitoring falls more to the client's level of responsibility. Health providers must discuss these topics frequently with their patients.

Oral medications

Before initiating additional pharmacologic therapy, it is essential to address the basics of the oral agent drug classifications for glucose control. First-generation sulfonylureas such as tolbutamide (Orinase), second-generation sulfonylureas such as glipizide (Glucotrol), and rapid-acting agents such as repaglinide (Prandin) all stimulate the pancreas to release insulin. However, these agents only address the cause of release, not that of insulin-receptor sensitivity. They also lower blood glucose levels by increasing the circulating insulin, which may cause early deterioration of beta cells.

α-Glucosidase inhibitors include acarbose (Precose) and miglitol (Glyset). α-Glucosidase inhibitors are metabolized by intestinal bacteria and digestive enzymes, delaying carbohydrate absorption in the gut. They are very appropriate for the individual who has normal fasting blood glucose levels and significantly elevated postprandial levels.

Before 1995, first and second generation sulfonylureas and rapid-acting agents such as repaglinide (Prandin) and nateglinide (Starlix) were the treatment of choice for patients who suffered from type 2 diabetes. These agents are quite effective in managing glucose levels, but do not address the cause of the irregularity. They lower the blood glucose levels by raising the insulin levels, which are already elevated, leading to possible beta cell failure and increasing the risk of hypoglycemia.

Metformin (Glucophage), approved in the United States in 1995, is the most widely prescribed oral agent for glucose control. Metformin reduces hepatic glucose output and increases glucose uptake. It also reduces insulin levels, which protects beta cells and reduces the risk of hypoglycemia [7].

Thiazolidinediones, including rosiglitazone (Avandia) and pioglitazone (Actos), act by increasing insulin-receptor sensitivity without stimulating insulin release. By increasing receptor sensitivity, more insulin is functional and less needs to be secreted by the beta cells, thus preserving beta cell function. Thiazolidinediones should be implemented early in oral diabetic pharmacologic management when patients are hyperinsulinemic [8].

The newer oral agents such as metformin and the thiazolidinediones better address the pathophysiologic causes of insulin and blood glucose problems. Rather than modifying just the blood glucose levels, the newer oral agents target the abnormal physiology. Some clinicians are still hesitant to institute these newer oral agents. However, early implementation of these agents in a patient's management plan can help maximize that patient's use of the insulin the body is still secreting.

Aspirin therapy

Aspirin therapy is recommended as primary prevention in patients aged 40 years and older who have diabetes and one or more cardiovascular risk factors. Use of aspirin has not been studied in diabetic individuals younger than 30 years. Low-dose aspirin therapy of 75 to 162 mg is recommended. Low-dose therapy has proved to be just as effective as higher doses in inhibiting thromboxane synthesis [9]. People who have aspirin allergy, bleeding tendency, recent gastrointestinal bleeding, clinically active hepatic disease, and are taking anticoagulant therapy are not candidates for aspirin therapy. Aspirin therapy is not recommended for patients younger than 21 years because of the increased risk of Reye's syndrome. Before aspirin therapy is initiated, it is imperative to control the client's blood pressure, or the risk of a hemorrhagic bleed significantly increases [10–13]. Box 3 lists risk factors for cardiovascular disease that should be considered before initiating aspirin therapy for patients who have diabetes.

Statin therapy

Individuals who suffer from diabetes are at the same high risk for a myocardial infarction (MI) as nondiabetic individuals who have had a previous MI. Patients who have coronary heart disease (CHD) and diabetes are at especially high risk for MIs; after the first MI, 1-year mortality rates in diabetic men are nearly twice as high as in nondiabetic men and 3.5-times as high in diabetic women compared with nondiabetic women [4]. Given the

---

Box 3. Cardiovascular risk factors suggestive for aspirin therapy

- Familial history of coronary heart disease
- Cigarette smoking
- Hypertension
- Obesity (>120% desirable weight); BMI >27.3 kg/m^2 in women, >27.8 kg/m^2 in men
- Albuminuria (micro or macro)
- Lipids:
  Cholesterol >180 mg/dL
  LDL cholesterol ≥100 mg/dL
  HDL cholesterol <45 mg/dL in men and <55 mg/dL in women
  Triglycerides >200 mg/dL
- Age >30 years

Abbreviations: BMI, body mass index; LDL, low-density lipoprotein; HDL, high-density lipoprotein.

From [25]. Clinical practice recommendations. Diabetes Care 2004;27(Suppl 1): S72–3; with permission.

---

well-understood association between cholesterol, CHD, and diabetes, close monitoring and control of cholesterol in diabetic clients is essential.

Along with blood pressure and glucose, the control and management of cholesterol is a targeted area of pharmacologic control. A low-density lipoprotein (LDL) level under 100 mg/dL is the primary goal. Secondary goals include triglyceride levels under 150 mg/dL and high-density lipoprotein (HDL) levels over 40 mg/dL in men and 50 mg/dL in women [3].

While other cholesterol-lowering agents (eg, fibric acid derivatives, nicotinic acid [niacin]) are available and in use, current trends promote the use of statins. Available statins include lovastatin, atorvastatin, gemfibrozil, and the new "super-statin" rosuvastatin. Rosuvastatin is hepatoselective, increases levels of HDL, and reduces levels of LDL, cholesterol, and triglycerides. A daily dosage of 10 to 40 mg has been shown to reduce LDL by 46% to 55% and increase HDL by 8% to 10%. Initial dosing is 10 mg per day titrating to the LDL goal. Monitoring of lipid levels should begin 2 to 4 weeks after initiation with dose titration. Aspartate aminotransferase (formerly called serum glutamic-oxaloacetic transaminase) and alanine aminotransferase (formerly called serum glutamic-pyruvic transaminase) should be monitored at baseline, 12 weeks, and 6 months. Significant consideration should be given to drug interactions, side effects, and contraindications of rosuvastatin. For example, levels of rosuvastatin increase 7 to 11 fold with cyclosporin, and concurrent use of antacids can reduce plasma concentrations by 54%. Dose-related increases in dipstick-positive proteinuria and microscopic hematuria have also been observed.

Use of rosuvastatin is contraindicated in active liver disease, during pregnancy, and with unexplained persistent elevations of serum transaminases. Rosuvastatin should be used cautiously in individuals who have a history of liver disease, high consumption of alcohol, and severe renal insufficiency (creatinine clearance under 30 mL/min). Rosuvastatin at dosages greater than 40 mg should be used cautiously in patients who have proteinuria and hematuria [7].

Ezetimibe (Zetia) is another relatively new statin. It inhibits absorption of cholesterol and localizes at the brush border of the small intestine. Ezetimibe has a half-life of 22 hours and achieves its maximal response within 2 weeks. The drug is used primarily in combination with other statins, yielding an LDL reduction of 46% to 58% in combination with simvastatin, and 53% to 61% in combination with atorvastatin. Ezetimibe can cause back pain, arthralgia, diarrhea, abdominal pain, and possible allergic reactions, and has drug interactions with gemfibrozil, fenofibrate, cyclosporin, and cholestyramine. A dosage of 10 mg per day can be taken with or without food, and shows no increased benefit with titration [7].

Angiotensin-converting enzyme inhibitor and angiotensin-receptor blocker therapies

Blood pressure in the diabetic client should be targeted at or below 130/80 mm Hg, according to the current recommendations of the ADA [3]. Initial therapy for hypertension should involve angiotension-converting enzyme (ACE) inhibitors, angiotension receptor blockers (ARBs), β-blockers, or diuretics. β-blockers should be used cautiously in patients with diabetes as a result of the block of sympathetic responses to hypoglycemia. Current, progressive management of diabetes mellitus in patients older than 55 years includes the addition of an ACE inhibitor to the pharmacologic therapy. These clients may or may not have hypertension, but possess other cardiovascular risk factors. Renal function declines progressively in clients who have diabetic nephropathy. This decline may be slowed by antihypertensive drugs, especially those with kidney-protecting properties [14]. The use of an ACE inhibitor reduces the risk of renal disease progression in patients suffering from the disease by 55% to 75% compared with patients who have normal renal function [15]. Increases in serum creatinine stabilize within the first 2 months of ACE inhibitor therapy.

ACE inhibitor therapy is indicated in patients who have diabetic nephropathy and in those who have nondiabetic nephropathies when protein excretion exceeds 1 g/dL. ACE inhibitor therapy should be discontinued temporarily if acute renal failure (ARF) evolves, and may be reinstituted once the ARF has been resolved. Hyperkalemia is a potential complication of ACE inhibitor therapy, particularly in clients who have diabetes or chronic renal failure. Therefore, early monitoring of serum potassium is warranted after therapy is initiated [16].

Use of an angiotensin-receptor blocker (ARB) significantly reduces the progression of nephropathy and conserves renal and cardiovascular function in patients who have diabetes [17–19]. Independent of their blood pressure–lowering effect, ARBs are considered to be renoprotective in patients who have type 2 diabetes and microalbuminuria, and therefore should be strongly considered for the management regimen.

Dual blockade effects

Many patients who have diabetic nephropathy have levels of albuminuria over 1 g/d and blood pressures over 135/85 mm Hg despite antihypertensive therapy. Such patients might benefit from dual blockade of the renin angiotensin system, which reduces albuminuria and blood pressure in patients who have type 2 diabetes. Specifically, a 25% mean reduction in albuminuria a 35% mean reduction in the fractional clearance of albumin, and a 10 mm Hg reduction in blood pressure are desirable [20].

Dual therapy with an ACE inhibitor and an ARB is recommended for those clients who require aggressive blood pressure control. Monitoring of the serum potassium levels is essential with this regimen. Maintenance of the serum potassium level below 5.6 mEq/L is important, with levels of 4.0 to 4.5 mEq/L considered ideal. Serum creatinine monitoring is also an important management strategy. A serum creatinine up to 20 mg/dL is acceptable, with an upward trend of 30 mg/dL or over considered alarming and cause for discontinuation of drug therapy. Correction of the fluid status should ensue following discontinuation, and pharmacologic therapy may be reinstituted after obtaining an initial creatinine baseline. Levels should be checked again at 2 weeks, and every few weeks thereafter. Maintaining adequate hydration of the patient undergoing dual therapy is extremely important [7].

Glucose controlling agents

Traditional management strategies remain in effect for glucose control along with the newer pharmacologic recommendations for controlling comorbid conditions. For type 2 diabetics, oral glucose-controlling agents are the first-line therapy. The biguanide metformin continues to be the most commonly used oral agent. The recommendation is to begin treatment at 500 mg/d and to titrate upwards to 850 to 1000 mg twice a day as needed. Metformin is currently the only oral agent shown to decrease vascular macular damage. It is approved for use in children aged 12 years and older [8].

Because glycemic control in patients deteriorates over time, oral combination therapy is often required. For those individuals who cannot maintain glycemic control on monotherapy, or whose hemoglobin A1C levels remain consistently under 7% on monotherapy, addition of a second oral agent may be beneficial. Combination oral therapy of metformin and the thiazolidinedione rosiglitazone has demonstrated a decrease in the mean

Table 2
Treatment algorithm for management of type 2 diabetes mellitus

Action	Goal
Patient education:	Glycemic control
Disease etiology	A1C <7%
Interventions	
Lifestyle modification	Preprandial plasma glucose
	90–130 mg/dL
Pharmacologic intervention	
Outcomes of diabetes mellitus	
Lifestyle modification:	Postprandial plasma
	glucose <180 mg/dL
Diet/nutrition	
Exercise	
Weight control	
Continue while effective, monitoring	
every 3 months	
If lifestyle modification is ineffective,	
begin monotherapy; while adequate,	
continue and monitor	
If monotherapy is inadequate, add a second	
oral agent; if dual therapy is adequate,	
monitor	
If dual therapy is inadequate:	
add bedtime insulin; or,	
add a third oral agent; or,	
switch to insulin monotherapy; and,	
consider referral to specialist	
Monitor A1C every 6 months in individuals	
who are at goal, and quarterly in those	
who are not at goal or who have had	
their therapy changed.	
Less intensive glycemic goals may be indicated	
in patients with severe or frequent hypoglycemia.	
Postprandial glucose may be targeted	
if A1C goals are not met despite	
reaching preprandial glucose goals.	
Monitor serum lipid levels.	LDL <100 mg/dL
	Triglycerides <150 mg/dL
	HDL >40 mg/dL in men
	HDL >50 mg/dL in women
If lipid levels are not at goal, consider a	
lipid-lowering agent.	
Monitor blood pressure.	<130/80 mm Hg
If BP not controlled, consider initial therapy with:	
ACE	
ACE alternatives	
ARBs	
β-blockers	
Diuretics	
For clients >55 y, with or without hypertension but	
with other CV risk factors, consider adding an ACE.	

(*continued on next page*)

Table 2 (*continued*)

Action	Goal
Consider aspirin therapy (75–162 mg/d) for clients ≥40 y with diabetes and one or more CV risk factors (ensure hypertension is controlled prior to initiating aspirin therapy).	
Monitor laboratory studies and physical signs and symptoms for altering responses and other disease effects.	

Abbreviations: LDL, low-density lipoprotein; HDL, high-density lipoprotein; BP, blood pressure; ACE, angiotension-converting enzyme; ARB, angiotension receptor blocker; CV, cardiovascular.

From American Diabetes Association. Clinical practice recommendations 2004. Diabetes Care 2004;(Suppl I):S1–73; with permission.

level of A1C—by 1% with 4 mg/d metformin-rosiglitazone dosing and 1.2% with 8 mg/d metformin-rosiglitazone dosing. This dual oral therapy improves glycemic control, insulin sensitivity, and beta-cell function more effectively than monotherapy [21].

Insulin therapy remains the pharmacologic agent of choice for type 1 diabetics and for type 2 diabetics whose insulin is insufficient in quantity or whose endogenous insulin has become ineffective at the receptor sites.

Summary

Diabetes is a chronic disease associated with multisystem complications. In particular, cardiovascular and renal demise are almost certain in individuals who have diabetes, with cardiovascular complications accounting for over 50% of mortality among patients who have type 2 diabetes mellitus [22]. Documented benefits of lowering cholesterol, blood pressure, and glucose levels in these patients have led to the current emphasis on multidimensional pharmacologic management. Table 2 provides a summary of recommendations for managing patients who have type 2 diabetes.

References

[1] Mokdad AH, Ford ES, Bowman BA, et al. Diabetes trends in the U.S.: 1990–1998. Diabetes Care 2000;23:1278–83.

[2] Bakris GL, Williams M, Dworkin L, et al. Preserving renal function in adults with hypertension and diabetes: a consensus approach. Am J Kidney Dis 2000;36(3):646–61.

[3] American Diabetes Association. Standards of medical care for patients with diabetes mellitus. Diabetes Care 2003;26(Suppl 1):S33–50.

[4] Rosenson RS. Lipoprotein-altering therapies to prevent cardiovascular disease in patients with type 2 diabetes. Prev Card Clinic. Sep 2003;3.

[5] Tanasescu M, Leitzmann MF, Rimm EB, et al. Physical activity in relation to cardiovascular disease and total mortality among men with type 2 diabetes. Circulation 2003;107:2435–9.

[6] Bickston TH. Medical-surgical nursing recall. Philadelphia: Lippincott Williams & Wilkins; 2004.

[7] Steadman S. New drug update 2003: a potpourri of new drugs, new warnings, and new indications. Paper presentation, 10th Annual Pharmacology in Advanced Practice Conference, Myrtle Beach, South Carolina, September 18–20 2003.

[8] Bartol TG. Treating type 2 diabetes to goal: the role of pharmacotherapy. Am J for NP 2003; 7(11):34–7.

[9] American Diabetes Association. Nutrition principles and recommendations in diabetes. Diabetes Care 2004;27(Suppl 1):S36–S46, S72–3.

[10] Colwell JA. Aspirin therapy in diabetes (technical review). Diabetes Care 1997;20:1767–71.

[11] Hansson L, Zanchetti A, Carruthers SG, et al. Effects of intensive blood-pressure lowering and low-dose aspirin in patients with hypertension: principle results of the Hypertension Optimal Treatment (HOT) randomized trial. Lancet 1998;351:1755–62.

[12] CAPRIE Steering Committee. A randomized, blinded trial of clopidogrel versus aspirin in patients at risk of ischaemic events (CAPRIE). Lancet 1996;348:1329–39.

[13] Peterson JG, Topol EJ, Sapp SK, et al. Evaluation of the effects of aspirin combined with angiotensin-converting enzyme inhibitors in patients with coronary artery disease. Am J Med 2000;109:371–7.

[14] Lewis EJ, Hunsicker LG, Bain RP, et al. The effect of angiotensin-converting enzyme inhibition on diabetic nephropathy. N Engl J Med 1993;329:1456–62.

[15] Bakris GL, Weir MR. Angiotensin-converting enzyme inhibitor-associated elevations in serum creatinine. Arch Intern Med 2000;160:685–93.

[16] Schoolwerth AC, Sica DA, Ballermann BJ, et al. Renal considerations in angiotensin converting enzyme inhibitor therapy: a statement for healthcare professionals from the Council on the Kidney in Cardiovascular Disease and the Council for High Blood Pressure Research of the American Heart Association. Circulation 2001;104:1985–91.

[17] Brenner BM, Cooper ME, Zeeuw DD, et al. Effects of losartan on renal and cardiovascular outcomes in patients with type 2 diabetes and nephropathy. N Engl J Med 2001;345:861–9.

[18] Lewis EJ, Hunsicker LG, Clarke WR, et al. Renoprotective effect of the angiotensin-receptor antagonist irbesartan in patients with nephropathy due to type 2 diabetes. N Engl J Med 2001;345:851–60.

[19] Parving HH, Lehnert H, Brochner-Mortensen J, et al. The effect of irbesartan on the development of diabetic nephropathy in patients with type 2 diabetes. N Engl J Med 2001; 345:870–8.

[20] Rossing K, Christensen PK, Jensen BR, et al. Dual blockade of the renin-angiotensin system in diabetic nephropathy: a randomized double-blind crossover study. Diabetes Care 2002;25: 95–100.

[21] Fonseca V, Rosenstock J, Patwardhan R, et al. Effect of metformin and rosiglitazone combination therapy in patients with type 2 diabetes mellitus. JAMA 2000;283:1695–702.

[22] Huang ES, Meigs JB, Singer DE. The effect of interventions to prevent cardiovascular disease in patients with type 2 diabetes mellitus. Am J Med 2001;111:633–42.

[23] American Diabetes Association. Physical activity/exercise and diabetes. Diabetes Care 2004; 27(suppl 1):S58–62.

[24] American Diabetes Association. Standards of medical care in diabetes. Diabetes Care 2004; 27(suppl 1):S15–35.

[25] American Diabetes Association. Clinical practice recommendations. Diabetes Care 2004; 27(suppl 1):S1–73.

NURSING
CLINICS
OF NORTH AMERICA

ELSEVIER
SAUNDERS

Nurs Clin N Am 40 (2005) 119–133

Osteoporosis: Incidence, Prevention, and Treatment of the Silent Killer

Lynn C. Parsons, DSN, RN, CNA

*School of Nursing, Box 81, Middle Tennessee State University,
Murfreesboro, TN 37132, USA*

Osteoporosis is a universal health crisis. Millions of American men and women are adversely affected by this disease as a result of increased longevity. Osteoporosis limits the ability to care for oneself independently and reduces the capacity to move about without fear of breaking a bone. In osteoporosis, bone becomes porous as a result of a decrease in bone density and the structural deterioration of bone tissue, which leads to bone weakness and vulnerability to fracture [1–3]. Osteoporosis is usually defined by bone mineral density (BMD) and the incidence of low-trauma fractures (eg, caused by coughing, rolling over in bed, bending to put on shoes) [4]. Osteopenia (ie, low bone mass), the precursor to osteoporosis, affects 34 million Americans.

According to the literature and related research, most men view osteoporosis as a disease attributable only to women and are surprised to discover how prevalent the disease is in men [1]. Osteoporosis is fast becoming a threat to national health and safety, affecting both men and women and all age and race groups.

Pathophysiology

Peak bone density is reached between the ages of 25 [5] and 30 [6]. Healthy bone (Fig. 1) is complex living tissue that provides structural support to muscle tissue, protects vital soft organs, and stores calcium needed to build strength and maintain bone density. When resorption of bone tissue by osteoclasts is greater than the buildup of bone by osteoblasts, bone demineralization occurs causing bone to become porous and resulting in osteoporosis (Fig. 2). After peak bone density is reached in young

---

E-mail address: lparsons@mtsu.edu (L.C. Parsons).

doi:10.1016/j.cnur.2004.09.001
nursing.theclinics.com

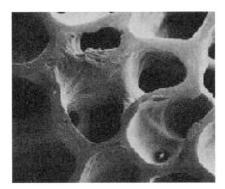

Fig. 1. Normal bone; normal findings on radiography. (Courtesy of the National Osteoporosis Foundation, Washington, DC, with permission.)

adulthood, a dual process of bone formation (ie, osteoblastic activity) and bone resorption (ie, osteoclastic activity) occurs, called remodeling.

Osteoporosis occurs as a result of a silent (ie, absence of symptoms) reduction of BMD, which can result in low-trauma fractures [2,7]. Frequently, patients discover that they have osteoporosis only after a fall that results in fracture.

Incidence

Common osteoporotic sites include the hip, spine, and wrist (Fig. 3) [8,9]. Spinal or vertebral fractures related to osteoporosis result in painful deformities and reduction in height. Hip fractures almost always require hospitalization and major surgery. Musculoskeletal injuries account for over 125 million lost workdays annually, resulting in a yearly cost of over $150 billion in lost wages and acute, chronic, and restorative health care admissions to hospitals, long-term care, and rehabilitation units [10].

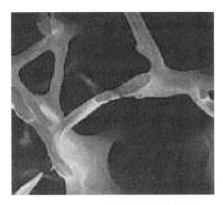

Fig. 2. Osteoporotic bone; abnormal findings on radiography. (Courtesy of the National Osteoporosis Foundation, Washington, DC, with permission.)

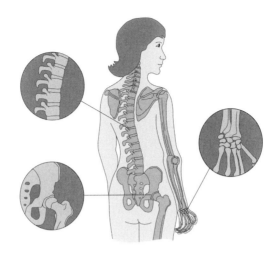

Fig. 3. Susceptible fracture sites related to osteoporosis: hip, spine, and wrist. (Courtesy of the National Osteoporosis Foundation, Washington, DC, with permission.)

Osteoporosis is a major health threat to approximately 44 million Americans [1]. The National Institute on Aging reports that 10 million Americans already have the disease, and another 34 million are at risk for osteoporosis as a result of low bone mass [9].

Osteoporosis is frequently viewed as an older person's disease, but it can strike at any age [11]. Osteoporosis is seen in young people when they fail to reach peak bone mass during childhood and adolescence. Age-related bone loss as a result of abrupt estrogen loss during menopause accounts for the increased prevalence of osteoporosis in women.

Gender differences

Women are affected by osteoporosis at a rate of four to one when compared with men [1,12]. Women are more vulnerable to osteoporosis because of the estrogen loss that occurs around menopause and the continued bone loss that occurs within 5 to 7 years following menopause. Men also have a larger and stronger skeleton than women, which partially explains why women are more prone to osteoporosis and osteoporosis-related fractures.

However, men are not immune to osteoporosis. More than 2 million American men suffer from osteoporosis [13], and another 3.5 million have osteopenia and are therefore at risk for developing the disease [14]. Close to 13% of men over the age of 50 will suffer an osteoporosis-related fracture. The mortality rate of older men who have hip fractures is increasing as a result of the improved longevity of Americans.

It is important for health care professionals to determine the osteoporosis knowledge-base for older men [5]. Because most men do not view this as a disease they will acquire, they need to be made aware of their susceptibility to the disease and measures they need to take for disease prevention. In a brochure circulated by the National Osteoporosis Foundation, the following statement summed up the way many men view this disease:

> I swung my golf club and felt intense pain in my back. The doctor at the hospital said I had a vertebral fracture from osteoporosis. Osteoporosis! I'm a 52-year-old healthy man, and I thought osteoporosis was a disease that affected older women! [13]

Research completed by Sedlak and colleagues [5] found that osteoporosis education was lacking for men. In this investigation, the men older than 65 years who were surveyed (N = 138) reported that they were confident to complete osteoporosis prevention strategies, but their performance of these behaviors was below recommended levels. Intake of daily dietary calcium was especially low for these men. Men need to become better educated about osteoporosis, health-promotion behaviors, and disease-prevention tactics through visits with their health practitioner and through community programs.

By 2040, the incidences of osteoporotic hip fractures could triple as a result of the growing number of geriatric patients [15]. Osteoporosis will be diagnosed in one in every three men over the age of 75. Men are experiencing a growing number of hip fractures, accounting for 25% of the annual incidences. Of the 100,000 men who sustain hip fractures, one third of them die within a year of the fracture [13]. While there continues to be national recognition of this disease in women, the impact of osteoporosis on men's health is often insufficiently researched, underdiagnosed, and inadequately reported.

Prevention and treatment

Living a healthy lifestyle and building strong bones, especially before the age of 30, is important in the prevention of osteoporosis. A diet that includes appropriate amounts of calcium and vitamin D is essential to achieving and maintaining peak bone mass [16]. Part of good bone health involves not smoking, low caffeine intake, and limited alcohol use. Smoking and alcohol consumption can have an adverse effect on BMD. Research supports that lower BMD is observed in the lumbar spine for patients who smoke [17].

Moderate weight-bearing and resistance exercises can prevent or modify bone density loss [18–20]. Simple activities such as mowing the lawn, raking, and weeding provide weight-bearing exercises (eg, pushing, pulling, digging) that help to preserve bone integrity. Exercises that specifically focus on weight-bearing and resistance training, such as those listed in Box 1, are recommended. These exercises, when used in combination with diet, vitamin supplements, and osteoporosis prevention and treatment medication, strengthen muscle and improve bone strength. Patients need to be informed that although swimming and bicycling are great forms of exercise for the cardiovascular system and promote a slimmer waistline, they are not considered weight-bearing exercises that promote good bone health.

BMD screening is the only sure way to determine bone density and fracture risk [21–23]. Those at risk for osteoporosis should have BMD testing. Box 2 lists factors to consider when assessing the risk for osteoporosis.

Certain disease processes contribute to risks associated with osteoporosis. A few examples include low testosterone production, some neoplastic diseases, steroid therapy, and gastric surgeries [24]. There are several tests to measure BMD and to determine bone health and fracture risk; all are noninvasive, pain free, and safe. Box 3 lists the different tests that a physician may order. BMD testing must be coupled with a full medical workup and the other measures for bone health promotion already outlined.

Vitamin and mineral therapy

Calcium is a primary mineral for maintaining bone density [25–29]. Foods rich in calcium, such as those listed in Box 4 are needed because the

---

Box 1. Exercise programs for osteoporosis prevention

Weight-bearing[a]
  Jogging
  Walking
  Stair climbing
  All types of dancing
  Soccer
  Ice/roller skating

Resistance training[b]
  Weight lifting[c]
  Full body workouts 2 to 3 times weekly, consisting of three sets
    of eight repetitions

---
  [a] Exercises where bone and muscle work against gravity.
  [b] Exercises including activities that improve muscle mass (density) and strengthen bone.
  [c] Especially metal weights. Bones need to lift weight to grow. Placing stress on the skeleton increases bone strength.

Box 2. Risk factors for osteoporosis

- History of fracture as an adult
- History of fracture in first-degree relatives (eg, parent, sibling)
- Current cigarette smoker
- High caffeine consumption
- Low body weight (<127 lbs)
- Female: Caucasian or Asian
- Early menopause
- Postmenopausal women, especially ages >65
- Women on prolonged hormone therapy
- Increased age
- Excessive alcohol consumption
- Sedentary lifestyle (little weight-bearing exercise)
- Inadequate dietary calcium and vitamin D intake
- Inadequate exposure to sunlight
- Medications to treat certain chronic illnesses (eg, hypothyroidism, seizure disorders, gastrointestinal diseases), especially the following:
  Excessive thyroid hormones
  Anticonvulsants
  Antacids containing aluminum
  Gonadotropin-releasing hormone used for treating endometriosis
  Methotrexate for cancer treatment
  Cyclosporine A (immunosuppressant)
  Heparin
  Cholestyramine

Data from refs. [21–23].

---

human body does not manufacture calcium. Calcium can be lost through diaphoresis (ie, sweat), hair, nails, and the constantly sloughing epidermal layer of the integumentary system. After the body has achieved complete skeletal growth, it is important to maintain adequate dietary intake of calcium in the diet or through calcium supplements (Table 1). An additional daily intake of 1000 mg of calcium is recommended to augment dietary calcium. Persons over the age of 51 are recommended to take 1200 mg to supplement their dietary calcium intake.

Vitamin D, which facilitates absorption of calcium into bone, is manufactured in the skin after direct exposure to direct sunlight [29]. Housebound individuals should be exposed to direct sunlight 10 to 15 minutes, two to three times a week with their hands, arms, and face exposed

---

Box 3. Types of Bone Mineral Density (BMD) Tests

There are several different machines that measure bone density. Central machines measure density in the hip, spine, and total body. Peripheral machines measure density in the finger, wrist, kneecap, shin bone, and heel.

DXA (dual energy x-ray absorptiometry): Measures the spine, hip, and total body

pDXA (peripheral dual energy x-ray absorptiometry): Measures the wrist, heel, and finger

SXA (single energy x-ray absorptiometry): Measures the wrist and heel

QUS (quantitative ultrasound): Uses sound waves to measure density at the heel, shin bone, and kneecap

QCT (quantitative computed tomography): Most commonly used to measure the spine, but can be used at other sites

pQCT (peripheral quantitative computed tomography): Measures the wrist

RA (radiographic absorptiometry): Uses an x-ray of the hand and a small metal wedge to calculate bone density

DPA (dual photon absorptiometry): Measures the spine, hip, and total body (used infrequently)

SPA (single photon absorptiometry): Measures the wrist (used infrequently)

Courtesy of the National Osteoporosis Foundation, Washington, DC, with permission.

---

for maximum benefit. Window glass, clothing, sunscreen, and air pollution inhibit exposure to sunlight and the manufacturing of vitamin D.

Major food sources of vitamin D include, but are not limited to, egg yolks, liver, salmon, cod liver oil, saltwater fish, and vitamin D-fortified dairy products such as milk and cheese. Vitamin D supplements are recommended in addition to dietary intake through food sources [30]. Nutritionists recommend between 400 and 800 daily IUs of vitamin D to maintain healthy bone.

Research has shows that inadequate intake of vitamin K may predispose elders to osteoporosis [30]. Foods rich in vitamin K, such as green leafy vegetables are important to bone health, osteoporosis prevention, and decreased fracture potential. Weight-bearing exercise, adequate intake of dietary calcium, and vitamins used in combination with osteoporosis prevention drug therapy all enhance bone health.

Box 4. Good sources of calcium

Low-fat milk
Cheese
Broccoli
Yogurt
Ice-cream
Tofu
Rhubarb
Almonds
Figs
Turnip greens
Canned salmon and sardines

Pharmacologic management

Adequate diet, exercise, and vitamin therapy in conjunction with drug management can slow bone loss. Most common forms of pharmacologic interventions include the bisphosphonates alendronate and risedronate, calcitonin, estrogens, parathyroid hormone, and raloxifene [31–33]. All of these medications decrease bone resorption and are approved by the Food and Drug Administration (FDA).

Alendronate is prescribed for the prevention or treatment of osteoporosis. Use of this drug decreases the incidence of osteoporosis-related spinal

Table 1
Recommended calcium intakes[a]

Ages	Amount mg/d
Birth–6 mo	210
6 mo–1	270
1–3	500
4–8	800
9–13	1300
14–18	1300
19–30	1000
31–50	1000
51–70	1200
≥70φ	1200
Pregnant & lactating	
14–18	1300
19–50	1000

National surveys have shown that many Americans are not consuming enough calcium. Many women, in fact, consume less than half of the daily recommended amount of calcium.
Courtesy of the National Osteoporosis Foundation, Washington, DC, with permission.
[a] Source: National Academy of Sciences.

and hip fractures by 50% [34]. According to the research literature, alendronate is one of the most frequently used medications to combat osteoporosis [35,36]. Alendronate may be taken daily or weekly (Table 2). Research completed by Walling [37] found comparable efficacy between daily and weekly dosing. Women tolerated the weekly treatment, fewer medication side effects were experienced, and it may be preferred to daily dosing because of the inconvenience of remaining without food or fluid for 30 minutes to an hour after administration [37].

Risedronate is the second major bisphosphonate to prevent and treat osteoporosis [34]. This medication lowers the risk of fractures in the hip and vertebrae by 30% to 40%. Additionally, when taken as a daily treatment, this medication increases BMD and decreases the risk of vertebral fracture within 1 year for men on corticosteroid therapy [38].

Raloxifene is a selective estrogen receptor modulator that prevents and treats osteoporosis [34]. This drug lowers the incidence of vertebral fractures by 40%. Research suggests that Raloxifene has positive effects on several markers of cardiac risk [39]. The ongoing research study Raloxifene Use for the Heart (RUTH) will not be completed until 2006; therefore, how it affects the overall markers of cardiac disease is yet to be determined.

Calcitonin is a polypeptide hormone that reduces the resorptive action of osteoclasts [34]. This medication may reduce the incidence of vertebral fractures by 35%. Research supports that 200 IU of nasal spray calcitonin taken daily is safe and effective in increasing lumbar BMD and reducing bone turnover in men with idiopathic osteoporosis [40].

Forteo, the newest medication being prescribed to treat osteoporosis [41–43], was approved by the FDA in November 2002. This drug is the first medication in a new class of bone-forming agents to actually stimulate the growth of new bone by increasing the action of osteoblasts. This injectable drug is administered once daily in the thigh or abdomen. Long-term safety is not known. Therefore, use of this medication is limited to no more than 2 years [44].

Bone growth increases BMD, which in turn decreases the susceptibility to fracture. Forteo contains parathyroid hormone, which is the primary regulator of calcium and phosphate metabolism in bones. There are several common drugs available that affect calcium levels and bone mineralization (see Table 2). Initial concern about Forteo was expressed by a consumer watchdog group called Public Citizen, which warned consumers that studies showed the drug caused a rare form of bone cancer in rats [45]. Cancer has not yet been identified in human subjects.

Caution must be exercised when taking anticonvulsants and other medications such as steroids, which are frequently prescribed for asthma, arthritis, and kidney disease, because they can weaken bone. Secondary osteoporosis is caused by medical treatments that decrease BMD [25]. One man wrote to the National Osteoporosis Foundation with the following comment: "I have severe asthma and have been on the medication,

Table 2
Common drugs affecting calcium levels and bone mineralization

Drug	Dose	Route	Mechanism of action	Adverse reactions and contraindicators	Special instructions
Raloxifene (Evista)	60 mg daily	PO	Preserves BMD and reduces plasma levels of cholesterol	Can cause deep vein thrombosis, hot flashes; FDA risk category X (the potential for fetal harm outweighs any possible benefit in pregnancy)	Take with or without food
Alendronate (Fosamax)	For osteoporosis prevention 5 mg daily 35 mg weekly For osteoporosis treatment 10 mg daily 70 mg weekly	PO	Decreases bone resorption by osteoclasts	Esophagitis; No other serious side effects	Take in the AM with a full glass of water, and before ingesting food or fluids (except water); remain upright (seated or standing) for at least 30 min, and after completing the first meal of the day.
Risedronate (Actone)	5 mg daily 35 mg weekly	PO	Decreases bone resorption by osteoclasts	Esophagitis, arthralgia, diarrhea, headache, rash, nausea	Take in the AM with a full glass of water, and before ingesting food or fluids (except water); remain upright (seated or standing) for at least 30 min, and after completing the first meal of the day.

Calcitonin–salmon nasal spray (Miacalcin)	100 IU; same for all routes	Nasal spray IM SQ	Prevention of osteoporosis	Nasal dryness and irritation	None; all routes are safe
Teriparatide (Forteo)[a]	20 µg daily	SQ	Increases BMD primarily by increasing bone deposition by osteoblasts	Nausea, headache, back pain, leg cramps; initial dosing may cause hypotension and associated vertigo	Avoid use in patients who have bone cancer or bone metastases

Abbreviations: IM, intramuscularly; SQ, subcutaneously.
[a] Eli Lilley is working on manufacturing Forteo in tablet, patches, and nasal spray administration routes.

prednisone for many years. This medication makes it easier for me to breathe, but I have developed severe osteoporosis as a result of using it." [13]

Additional literature and related research

A review of the available literature indicates that osteoporosis prevention and treatment is vastly underresearched. Of the 102 research studies in the United States and other countries, 96% of them were published in medical journals and focused on pharmacologic interventions [46–48]. This was followed by 2% in nutrition journals, 1% in nursing journals, and 1% in pharmacology journals [49,50].

Seven data-based investigations studied aspects of osteoporosis and fracture prevention, including exercise, diet, physician role, environmental factors (eg, safety), untimely diagnosis, cessation of smoking, and reduced alcohol consumption [51,52]. Underfoot accidents in the home (eg, tripping on a rug) were frequent causes of osteoporotic-related fractures for elders. Referrals from hospital nurses for home health care agencies are needed for patients' follow-up care and internal and external home assessment to determine environmental safety. A comparison study was done between a group of orthopaedic surgeons and a group of family practice physicians to determine which group should provide follow-up care and patient teaching following hospitalization for orthopaedic surgery. There was overwhelming agreement by both groups of physicians that family practitioners should provide this service to patients.

A survey of a group of elderly subjects (N = 145) revealed that 54% of the men knew that osteoporosis could affect them, but the women had more awareness of osteoporosis and were taking more calcium supplements than the men ($P < 0.001$) [53]. This study exposed the significant knowledge gaps within that representative group. Physicians ranked fifth as a source of information for these individuals.

Economics of osteoporosis

Caucasian females have a 50% likelihood of experiencing an osteoporosis-related fracture in their lifetime [44]. However, men also need to be cognizant of the adverse effects of osteoporosis. In the mid-1990s, more than 432,000 hospitalizations, approximately 2.5 half million office visits, and 180,000 admissions to long-term care facilities occurred as a result of osteoporosis and osteoporosis-related fractures. In 2001, the annual cost of these events was estimated at $17 billion, with a single hip fracture costing approximately $40,000 per hospitalization. The number of hip fractures, the associated costs, and the increasing longevity of Americans could more than triple by the year 2040.

Medications to treat osteoporosis are expensive. Forteo costs approximately $20/day and $7,000 annually [32]. The website, http://www.walgreens.com provides current costs of such medications at one widely used retailer [54]. Ten milligram tablets of Fosamax in a quantity of 30 costs approximately $70, 30 mg tablets of Actonel in a quantity of 30 costs approximately $530, 200 IU/mL of injectable calcitonin costs approximately $48, and 60 mg tablets of Evista in a quantity of 30 costs approximately $70. It is imperative that nurses educate patients about how these medications should be taken for maximum effectiveness (see Table 2).

Summary

Osteoporosis is a nationwide health care concern affecting millions of Americans. Health care dollars to prevent and treat osteoporosis are needed. Osteoporosis-related injuries and resulting disabilities, and consequent admissions to hospitals, nursing homes, and long-term care facilities is costing billions of dollars for care and treatment.

Healthy lifestyle choices including vitamin and mineral therapy; safe home environments; a diet replete with calcium, vitamin D, and protein; weight-bearing and resistance exercises; and fall prevention programs for home-bound and hospitalized elders are needed to prevent osteoporosis-related fractures and injuries. Nurses must educate the public on osteoporosis and osteoporosis-prevention activities.

Research in nursing, pharmacy, and allied health fields such as physical therapy and nutrition must expand to improve understanding of the risks associated with osteoporosis and to evaluate health-promotion and disease-prevention activities. Interdisciplinary partnerships should be established to study the issues, prevention, and treatment modalities of this "silent killer."

References

[1] National Osteoporosis Foundation (NOF). Disease statistics. Washington, DC: National Osteoporosis Foundation; 2004.
[2] Lawson MT. Evaluating and managing osteoporosis in men. Nurse Pract 2001;26:26–49.
[3] Lane JM, Khan SN, Diwan AD. Osteoporosis: current clinical trends. Clin Geriatr 2000;8: 27–39.
[4] Geier KA. Osteoporosis in men. Orthop Nurs 2001;20:49–56.
[5] Sedlak CA, Doheny MO, Estok PJ. Osteoporosis in older men: knowledge and health beliefs. Orthop Nurs 2000;19:38–46.
[6] National Osteoporosis Foundation (NOF). Osteoporosis—bone health. Washington, DC: National Osteoporosis Foundation; 2004.
[7] National Osteoporosis Foundation (NOF). Osteoporosis—what is it? Washington, DC: National Osteoporosis Foundation; 2004.
[8] Melton LJ III. The prevalence of osteoporosis: gender and racial comparison. Calcif Tissue Int 2001;69:179–81.
[9] Lewis C. Osteoporosis and men. FDA Consum 2002;36:15–8.

[10] Parsons LC, Krau SD, Ward KS. Orthopaedic trauma: managing secondary medical problems. Crit Care Nurs Clin N Am 2001;13:433–42.

[11] Moon MA. Be aware that osteoporosis also affects young women and men. Fam Pract News 2000;30:25–9.

[12] Taylor JR, Sicard D. What pharmacists should know about osteoporosis. Drug Topics 2003; 147:78–93.

[13] National Osteoporosis Foundation (NOF). Men with osteoporosis in their own words. Washington DC: National Osteoporosis Foundation; 2000.

[14] Harvard Men's Health Watch. Osteoporosis in men, Harv Mens Health Watch 1999;3(7): 1–4.

[15] Crandall C. Gender differences in osteoporosis treatment: a review of clinical research. J Gend Specif Med 2000;3:42–6.

[16] Hisel TM, Phillips BB. Update on the treatment of osteoporosis. Formulary 2003;38:223–39.

[17] Egger P, Duggleby S, Hobbs R, et al. Cigarette smoking and bone mineral density in the elderly. J Epidemiol Community Health 1996;50:47–50.

[18] National Osteoporosis Foundation (NOF). Prevention—exercise for healthy bones. Washington, DC: National Osteoporosis Foundation; 2004.

[19] Spiker T. Skeleton key: As you read this, your bones are becoming shorter, thinner, and more brittle. Do you know how to stop the decline? Men's Health 2002;17:88–91.

[20] Compston J. Secondary causes of osteoporosis in men. Calcif Tissue Int 2001;69:193–5.

[21] National Osteoporosis Foundation (NOF). Osteoporosis—bone mass measurement. Washington, DC: National Osteoporosis Foundation; 2004.

[22] Crandall C. Osteoporosis in men: where do we stand with screening and treatment. Consultant 2002;42:112–9.

[23] Wisewell RA, Hawkins SA, Dreyer HC, et al. Maintenance of BMD in older male runners is independent of changes in training volume or VO(2) peak. J Gerontol A Biol Sci Med 2002; 57:203–8.

[24] Baskin ST. Osteoporosis: some new diagnostic and treatment options. Cleveland Nursing Weekly, May 13, 1996.

[25] Ebeling PR, Wark JD, Yeung S, et al. Effects of calcitrol or calcium on bone mineral density, bone turnover, and fractures in men with primary osteoporosis: a two-year randomized, double blind, double placebo study. J Clin Endocrinol Metab 2001;86:4098–103.

[26] Rodriguez-Martinez MA, Garcia-Cohen EC. Role of Ca (2+) and vitamin D in the prevention and treatment of osteoporosis. Pharmacol Ther 2002;93:37–49.

[27] National Osteoporosis Foundation (NOF). Prevention—who's at risk? Washington, DC: National Osteoporosis Foundation; 2004.

[28] National Osteoporosis Foundation (NOF). Prevention—calcium supplements. Washington, DC: National Osteoporosis Foundation; 2004.

[29] National Osteoporosis Foundation (NOF). Prevention—Calcium and Vitamin D. Washington, DC: National Osteoporosis Foundation; 2004.

[30] Tse SL, Chan TY, Wu DM, et al. Deficient dietary vitamin K intake among elderly nursing home residents in Hong Kong. Asia Pac J Clin Nutr 2002;11:62–5.

[31] National Osteoporosis Foundation (NOF). Medications—to prevent and treat osteoporosis. Washington, DC: National Osteoporosis Foundation; 2004.

[32] Lehne RA. Pharmacology for nursing care. 5th edition. Boston, MA: Saunders; 2004.

[33] Gutierrez K, Queener SF. Pharmacology for nursing practice. St. Louis, MO: Mosby; 2003.

[34] National Osteoporosis Foundation (NOF). Physician's guide to prevention and treatment of osteoporosis. Washington, DC: National Osteoporosis Foundation; 2003.

[35] Adami S, Prizzi R, Colapietro F. Alendronate for the treatment of osteoporosis in men. Calcif Tissue Int 2001;69:239–41.

[36] Ringe JD, Faber H, Dorst A. Alendronate treatment of established primary osteoporosis in men: results of a 2-year prospective study. J Clin Endocrinol Metab 2001;86:5252–5.

[37] Walling AD. Weekly therapy is effective in prevention of osteoporosis. Am Fam Physician 2003;68:1212–3.
[38] Reid DM, Adami S, Devogelaer JP, Chines AA. Risedronate increases bone density and reduces vertebral fracture risk within one year in men on corticosteroid therapy. Calcif Tissue Int 2001;69:242–7.
[39] Johnson K. Consider raloxifene a safe alternative to HRT. Family Practice News 2000;30: 27–30.
[40] Trovas GP, Lyritis GP, Galanos A, et al. A randomized trial of nasal spray salmon calcitonin in men with idiopathic osteoporosis: effects on bone mineral density and bone markers. J Bone Miner Res 2002;17:521–7.
[41] National Osteoporosis Foundation (NOF). National Osteoporosis Foundation comments on FDA approval of Forteo®. Washington, DC: National Osteoporosis Foundation; 2004.
[42] National Osteoporosis Foundation (NOF). Statement of the National Osteoporosis Foundation regarding FDA Committee's recommended approval of Forteo™. Washington, DC: National Osteoporosis Foundation; 2004.
[43] LoBuona C. New osteoporosis drug is first to form bone. Drug Topics 2003;147:24–5.
[44] National Osteoporosis Foundation (NOF). Pocket guide to prevention and treatment of osteoporosis. Washington DC: National Osteoporosis Foundation; 2003.
[45] Johnson K. Watchdog group issues warning against osteoporosis drug: expert questions legitimacy of claims. Family Practice News 2003;33:6–10.
[46] Brunk D. Studies conflict on gastrointestinal event risk from bisphosphonates: alendronate vs. risedronate. Internal Medicine News 2003;3:21–2.
[47] Campion JM, Maricic MJ. Osteoporosis in men. Am Fam Physician 2003;67:1521–30.
[48] Kanis JA, Johnell O, Oden A, et al. Diagnosis of osteoporosis and fracture threshold in men. Calcif Tissue Int 2001;69:218–21.
[49] Kim KK, Horan ML, Gendler P, et al. Development and evaluation of the osteoporosis health belief scale. Res Nurs Health 1991;14:155–63.
[50] Canty GH, Conde F, Rutledge DN. Osteoporosis in men treated with androgen suppression therapy for prostate cancer. Clinical Journal of Oncology Nursing 2002;6:88–103.
[51] Long D. Optimism for black men, women osteoporosis, and cancer sufferers. Diagnostic & Imaging Week 2002;5:1–2.
[52] Binkley NC, Suttie JW. Vitamin K nutrition and osteoporosis. J Nutr 1995;125:1812–22.
[53] Juby AG, Davis P. A prospective evaluation of the awareness, knowledge, risk factors and current treatment of osteoporosis in a cohort of elderly subjects. Osteoporos Int 2001;12: 617–22.
[54] Drug Information and Prices. Available at: http://www.walgreens.com. Accessed January 19, 2004.

ELSEVIER
SAUNDERS

NURSING
CLINICS
OF NORTH AMERICA

Nurs Clin N Am 40 (2005) 135–148

Emerging Trends in the Management of Heart Failure: Beta Blocker Therapy

Jenny L. Sauls, DSN, RN, C[a],*, Tom Rone, RN, CCRN[b]

[a]School of Nursing, Box 81, Middle Tennessee State University, Murfreesboro, TN 37132, USA
[b]Intensive Care Unit, Middle Tennessee Medical Center, 400 North Highland Avenue, Murfreesboro, TN 37130, USA

Heart failure continues to be a major health concern in the United States and accounts for approximately three million hospitalizations each year. An estimated five million people are affected by this debilitating disease [1] and despite advances in medical and surgical interventions, the death rate is 50% within five years of diagnosis [2,3]. This mortality rate results in 300,000 deaths annually [1]. As heart failure continues to be one of the most common reasons for hospitalization, the search continues for more effective treatment. Although historically the use of beta blocker therapy has not been recommended because of the negative inotropic effects, recent clinical trials indicate an actual reduction in mortality with the use of these drugs in the treatment of heart failure. Other added benefits include decreased numbers of hospitalizations, improvement of symptoms, and increased quality of life.

The purpose of this article is to review the pathophysiology of heart failure, and includes a brief discussion of compensatory mechanisms and clinical manifestations. A literature review is presented of clinical trials related to beta blocker therapy, actions of beta blockers, side effects, drug interactions, costs associated with beta blocker therapy, and, finally, nursing implications associated with administration of beta blockers.

Pathophysiology of heart failure

Heart failure, most commonly caused by coronary heart disease and hypertension, is defined as the heart's inability to meet the oxygenation

* Corresponding author.
  E-mail address: jsauls@mtsu.edu (J.L. Sauls).

needs of the body as a result of systolic or diastolic dysfunction [4]. Systolic dysfunction prohibits the heart's contractile ability, thereby limiting the forward flow of blood, whereas diastolic dysfunction inhibits the heart's ability to relax and fill with blood. The focus of this article is limited to systolic dysfunction. The end result of systolic dysfunction is a decrease in cardiac output, which leads to a series of compensatory mechanisms that ultimately result in cardiac decompensation. The major compensatory events involved in heart failure include sympathetic nervous system response, activation of the renin-angiotensin-aldosterone response, cardiac hypertrophy, and activation of natriuretic peptides [3–8].

Sympathetic nervous system response

When cardiac output falls, the sympathetic nervous system is activated within minutes, stimulating an increase in circulating levels of catechol-amines, primarily norepinephrine. This response results in an increase in heart rate, force of contraction, cardiac output, systemic vascular resistance, cardiac workload, and myocardial oxygen consumption. Short-term benefits include perfusion of vital organs and compensation for a decreased cardiac output. However, long-term activation of the sympathetic nervous system results in decompensation with resulting manifestations of heart failure and an increased mortality. Although cardiac output may initially be increased by this series of events, eventually it places a greater burden on an already failing heart and leads to decompensation [3–6,8].

Renin-angiotensin-aldosterone system

When the juxtaglomerular cells in the afferent arteriole of the kidney detect a decrease in perfusion as a result of a decreased cardiac output, renin is released and the renin-angiotensin-aldosterone system (RAAS) is initiated. Renin activates angiotensin, which causes vasoconstriction, and aldosterone, which causes sodium and water retention. Vasoconstriction leads to increased preload and afterload, whereas sodium and water retention lead to increased preload, all of which increase cardiac workload and oxygen consumption, again resulting in decompensation of a weakened heart [8].

Myocardial hypertrophy

To compensate for an increase in workload as a result of increased pressure or volume, the myocardium becomes hypertrophied. Pressure overload results in an increase in cell size and number, causing the myocardium to become thicker. Volume overload causes the myocytes to elongate, resulting in ventricular dilatation. This ventricular remodeling occurs in an attempt to maintain cardiac output. However, as the heart continues to enlarge and scar tissue develops, ischemia occurs and oxygen demands increase with an already failing myocardium, resulting in cardiac decompensation [3,8].

Natriuretic peptides

Two other hormones secreted in heart failure include atrial natriuretic peptide (ANP) and B-type natriuretic peptide (BNP). ANP, secreted by atrial cells in response to increased atrial filling pressures or atrial stretch, seems to inhibit the RAAS, thus having a diuretic and vasodilating effect [6]. BNP is a hormone secreted by ventricular cells in response to increased ventricular filling pressure or stretch. Like ANP, BNP has diuretic and vasodilating effects. BNP has been identified as a highly sensitive and specific serum marker for diagnosing heart failure and is said to presently be the most accurate diagnostic tool for identifying the presence and severity of heart failure [7].

The net effects of these compensatory mechanisms result in the clinical manifestations that may be observed in heart failure. Heart failure is classified as either left or right ventricular failure to enable easier understanding of the symptoms. Manifestations of left ventricular failure are associated with symptoms of respiratory compromise (eg, increased pulmonary venous pressure), and right ventricular failure results in systemic complications (eg, increased systemic venous pressure). Manifestations associated with left ventricular failure include dyspnea, fatigue, crackles on auscultation of breath sounds, tachycardia, arrhythmias, confusion, restlessness, weak peripheral pulses, cool extremities, and cough. Right ventricular failure results in peripheral edema, liver engorgement, jugular venous distention, ascites, weight gain, anorexia, nausea, and nocturia. As left ventricular failure is the most common cause of right ventricular failure, a mixture of left and right clinical manifestations may be exhibited [9].

Beta blockers

Beta blockers may be classified as either selective or nonselective. Selective beta-adrenergic blocking drugs inhibit the actions of β_1 receptors in the heart. Nonselective beta blockers inhibit β_1, β_2, and alpha receptors. β_2 receptors are located in the smooth muscles of the bladder, gastrointestinal tract, uterus, liver, bronchioles, and skeletal blood vessels. Alpha receptors are located in the liver, bladder sphincter, and muscles of the eyes, skin, and arterioles [10,11].

Administration of beta blockers inhibits actions of alpha and beta receptors, which decreases the detrimental effects of long-term activation of the sympathetic nervous system. Blockage of β_1 receptors slows heart rate and decreases speed of atrioventricular conduction and force of contraction, thereby decreasing the workload of the heart and oxygen consumption. When β_2 receptors are blocked, constriction of smooth muscles in the bronchioles, gastrointestinal tract, and bladder may occur. Blockage of alpha receptors result in dilation of arterioles; relaxation of the bladder sphincter, eye, and skin muscles; increased insulin secretion; and dilation of skeletal muscle vessels [8,10–12]. The most beneficial long-term effects of beta blocker therapy in heart failure include increased stroke volume and cardiac output; increased ejection fraction; decreased right and left heart pressures; decreased heart rate; and decreased systemic vascular resistance. These effects result in increased exercise tolerance, improvement of symptoms, and increased quality of life and overall well-being [11,13,14].

There are essentially three different types of beta blockers that have been evaluated for use in the management of heart failure: (1) cardioselective beta blockers that inhibit β_1 receptors (eg, metoprolol), (2) nonselective beta blockers that inhibit β_1 and β_2 activity (eg, propranolol), and (3) drugs that inhibit both alpha and beta receptor activity (eg, carvedilol) [11,12]. The most recent and extensive study is related to metoprolol and carvedilol.

Clinical trials

The Cardiac Insufficiency Bisoprolol Study II (CIBIS II) included 2647 participants from multiple sites in a double-blind randomized placebo-controlled trial. The participants were randomly assigned to one of two groups. Participants in the experimental group received bisoprolol in progressively increasing increments to a maximum dose of 10 mg per day, and participants in the control group received a placebo. All participants involved in the study were classified as New York Heart Association Class III or IV (indicating moderate or severe symptoms) heart failure with ejection fractions of 35% or less with a therapeutic regimen of diuretics and angiotensin-converting enzyme inhibitors [15].

Early results were so compelling that the study was terminated prematurely. Mortality in the experimental group was significantly less than the control group (11.8% versus 17.3%) regardless of the severity or cause of heart failure. Not only was mortality reduced with bisoprolol but the number of participants who were hospitalized was also significantly reduced, indicating a decrease in morbidity especially for worsening heart failure [15].

Another large-scale clinical trial, the Metoprolol CR/XL Randomized Intervention Trial in Congestive Heart Failure (MERIT-HF) study, was conducted to ascertain whether metoprolol would lower mortality in patients who had reduced ejection fraction and symptoms of heart failure when given primarily angiotensin converting enzyme (ACE) inhibitors and diuretics in addition to standard therapy. Other drug therapy taken by participants in this study included angiotensin receptor blockers, digitalis, aspirin, and lipid-lowering agents. This multi-site, double-blind, randomized controlled study included 3991 patients diagnosed with stable chronic heart failure New York Heart Association (NYHA) Class II, III, or IV(indicating mild, moderate, or severe symptoms), with ejection fractions of 40% or less. The patients were assigned to either the experimental group or the control group. Patients in the experimental group received standard therapy (specific to the individual) in addition to metoprolol in doses that were up-titrated over an eight-week period to a target dose of 200 mg once daily. Patients in the control group received a placebo in addition to their standard therapy [16].

Once again, results were so compelling that the study was terminated prematurely. Findings indicated a decrease in mortality from all causes, including worsening heart failure and sudden death, in patients receiving metoprolol. With a 38% decrease in mortality, the results of this study closely parallel the results of the CIBIS II trial in which there was a 34% decrease. The major difference between the two studies relates to death from worsening heart failure, which was decreased by 49% in the MERIT-HF trial and by only 26% in the CIBIS II trial. However, the CIBIS II trial did not include patients in NYHA Class II. Additionally, whereas the MERIT-HF study included patients who had an ejection fraction of 40% or less, the CIBIS II trail included patients who had ejection fraction of 35% or less [16]. Therefore, it might be concluded that patients in the CIBIS II trial were sicker initially than the patients in the MERIT-HF group, possibly explaining the difference in percentage of deaths resulting from worsening heart failure.

The MERIT-HF group was also evaluated for clinical deterioration or adverse events during the first 90 days. Results indicated that metoprolol was well-tolerated in patients diagnosed with NYHA Class II–IV stable chronic heart failure. Few adverse events were reported relating to blood pressure, heart rate, early discontinuation of drug, delayed titration, diuretic dosing, dosing of ACE inhibitors, breathlessness, or fatigue. This evidence indicates that beta blockers can be safely administered to patients who have heart failure [17].

In another double-blind randomized clinical trial, carvedilol was evaluated for effects on mortality and hospitalization. A group of 2289 patients who had severe heart failure and ejection fractions of less than 25% were assigned to either the experimental or the placebo group. Those in the experimental group received carvedilol in addition to standard therapy, which included diuretics and ACE inhibitors or angiotensin receptor blockers (ARBs). This study was also terminated prematurely because benefits became apparent approximately 10 months into the study. When compared with the placebo group, patients in the carvedilol group had a 35% lower mortality rate and a 24% lower combined risk of death and hospitalization. Also, fewer patients in the carvedilol group withdrew as a result of adverse reactions [11].

The Carvedilol or Metoprolol European Trial enlisted 3029 patients who had chronic heart failure. These patients were randomly assigned to either the carvedilol treatment group or the metoprolol treatment group. The purpose of this study was to compare the effects of carvedilol and metoprolol on morbidity and mortality. Patients who had chronic heart failure NYHA Class II–IV, prior cardiac history, ejection fraction less than 35%, and were currently undergoing treatment with diuretics and ACE inhibitors were included in the study. The findings of this study, which took place over approximately 58 months, revealed that mortality from all causes was 34% in the carvedilol group and 40% in the metoprolol group, suggesting that carvedilol extends survival longer when compared with metoprolol. Carvedilol extended survival by approximately 8 years and metoprolol extended survival by 6.6 years [18].

Another study comparing carvedilol and metoprolol included 150 patients who had heart failure NYHA Class II–IV and ejection fractions of 35% or less. All patients were also receiving furosemide and ACE inhibitors or ARBs. In the double-blind randomized trial, the patients were assigned to either the carvedilol or metoprolol group. Findings of the study showed that after 13 to 15 months of treatment, patients in the carvedilol group had greater increases in ejection fraction at rest and stroke volume during exercise. There was also a decrease in left heart pressures at rest and during exercise. Patients in the metoprolol group had greater exercise tolerance, although both drugs improved symptoms and quality of life to a similar degree. The differences in outcome for these drugs was linked to greater antiadrenergic activity of carvedilol compared with metoprolol, because carvedilol blocks both alpha and beta receptor activity [19].

Occurrence of adverse reactions in this last study was quite low. Worsening heart failure with up-titration of metoprolol was observed in 13 patients (17.3%), dizziness was noted in one patient (1.3%), and hypotension and symptomatic bradycardia were each observed in only two patients (2.7%). Adverse reactions to carvedilol included dizziness in 11 patients (14.7%), worsening heart failure in six patients (8%), symptomatic bradycardia in three patients (4%), hypotension in two patients (2.7%), and Raynaud's phenomenon in only one patient (1.3%) [19].

The Beta-Blocker Evaluation of Survival Trial was a double-blind, randomized study that recruited 2708 patients to participate in the evaluation of the effectiveness of bucindolol in decreasing mortality. After approximately two years of investigation, the study was terminated because no difference was observed between the bucindolol group and the placebo group. Adverse reactions that occurred with greater frequency in the bucindolol group were bradycardia, intermittent claudication, diarrhea, dizziness, and hyperglycemia [20].

In addition to the clinical trials just reviewed, a meta-analysis of 18 double-blind, placebo-controlled, randomized trials conducted before 1998 that encompassed 3023 patients showed that the use of beta blockers in patients who had heart failure decreased mortality and hospitalization by 37% and increased ejection fraction by 29% [21].

Even though there is overwhelming evidence that beta blockers decrease morbidity and mortality, these drugs remain underused in clinical practice for the treatment of heart failure. Physicians are concerned that the initiation and maintenance of therapy are difficult and may produce initial worsening of heart failure for as long as four to eight weeks. This concern, coupled with the delay in positive benefits of therapy, contributes to the current underuse of beta blockers for treatment of heart failure [22].

The Carvedilol Prospective Randomized Cumulative Survival Study (COPERNICUS), a large randomized, double-blind, controlled clinical trial was conducted for the purpose of evaluating early effects of beta blocker therapy in patients who had severe heart failure. This study included 2289 participants from multiple sites who were randomly assigned to one of two groups. Those assigned to the experimental group received carvedilol in progressively increasing increments up to a maximum dose of 25 mg twice daily, and participants in the control group received a placebo. All participants also received their usual medications for heart failure. Criteria for inclusion in the study required that all participants be symptomatic with minimal exertion or at rest, with an ejection fraction of less than 25% [22].

Results of the COPERNICUS study again indicate that mortality is decreased along with hospitalizations. Worsening of heart failure occurred with similar frequency in both groups: 6.4% in the placebo group and 5.1% in the group that received carvedilol. Positive results with carvedilol began to occur as early as 14 days after initial treatment. The study showed that initial benefit versus risk was similar to that for long-term therapy. The results of these trials should provide physicians with sufficient information to warrant using beta blocker therapy in treating heart failure [22].

Of the clinical trials reviewed, studies involving more that 17,000 patients support the use of beta blocking drugs in the treatment of heart failure. All trials evaluating metoprolol and carvedilol showed positive results related to morbidity and mortality. Only one study involving bucindolol showed no improvement relating to either morbidity or mortality. Studies comparing metoprolol and carvedilol revealed that carvedilol extends survival longer and has a greater positive impact on ejection fraction, and metoprolol has a more positive effect on exercise tolerance.

Nursing implications

Nurses must be aware of administration procedures, expected benefits of beta blocker therapy, adverse reactions (Table 1), financial burden (Table 2), and contraindications (Table 3) [23,24]. The positive effects of therapy have been discussed, but sometimes there are negative responses that nurses must be alert to in providing care for the patients who receive these drugs. Ongoing assessment and evaluation of possible adverse reactions is a responsibility

Table 1
Beta blocker adverse drug reactions

	Metoprolol	Carvedilol
> 10% of cases		
CNS	Drowsiness, insomnia	Dizziness, fatigue
Endocrine & metabolic	Decreased sexual ability	Hyperglycemia, weight gain
GI	—	Diarrhea
Neuromuscular & skeletal	—	Weakness
Respiratory	—	Upper respiratory tract infection
1% to 10% of cases		
Cardiovascular	Bradycardia, palpitations, edema, CHF, reduced peripheral circulation	Bradycardia, hypotension, AV block, angina, postural hypotension, syncope, dependent edema, palpitations, peripheral edema, generalized edema
CNS	Mental depression	Pain, headache, fever, paresthesia, somnolence, insomnia, malaise, hypesthesia, vertigo
Endocrine & metabolic	—	Gout, hypocholesteremia, dehydration, hyperkalemia, hypervolemia, hypertriglyceridemia, hyperuricemia, hypoglycemia, hyponatremia
GI	Diarrhea or constipation, nausea, vomiting, stomach discomfort	Nausea, vomiting, melena, periodentitis
Hematologic	—	Thrombocytopenia, decreased prothrombin, purpura
Hepatic	—	Increased transaminases, increased alkaline phosphatase
Neuromuscular & skeletal	—	Back pain, arthralgia, myalgia, muscle cramps
Ocular	—	Blurred vision
Renal	—	Increased BUN, abnormal renal function, albuminuria, glycosuria, increased creatinine, kidney failure

Respiratory	Bronchospasm	Sinusitis, bronchitis, pharyngitis, rhinitis, increased cough
Miscellaneous	Cold extremities	Infection, injury, increased diaphoresis, viral infection, allergy, sudden death
< 1% of cases		
Miscellaneous	Limited to important or life-threatening	Limited to important or life-threatening
	Arrhythmias, chest pain, confusion (especially in elderly), depression, dyspnea, hallucinations, headache, hepatic dysfunction, hepatitis, jaundice, leucopenia, nervousness, orthostatic hypotension, thrombocytopenia	Aggravated depression, anaphylactoid reaction, anemia, aplastic anemia (rare, all events occurred in patients receiving other medications capable of causing this effect), asthma, AV block (complete), bronchospasm, bundle branch block, convulsion, diabetes mellitus, exfoliative dermatitis, GI hemorrhage, leucopenia, migraine, myocardial ischemia, neuralgia, pancytopenia, peripheral ischemia, pulmonary edema, Stevens-Johnson syndrome

Abbreviations: AV, atrioventricular; BUN, blood urea nitrogen; CHF, congestive heart failure; CNS, central nervous system; GI, gastrointestinal.
Data from Lacey, CF, Armstrong LL, Goldman MP, et al. Drug information handbook, 10th edition Ohio: Lexi-Comp.; 2002.

Table 2
Cost comparison of beta blockers

Drug	Fill	Price
Metoprolol (Lopressor)	60 tabs (100 mg)	$11.99
	60 tabs (50 mg)	$10.99
Carvedilol (Coreg)	60 tabs (6.25 mg, 12.5 mg, 25 mg)	$110.99
Bisoprolol (Zebeta)	30 tabs (10 mg)	$52.99

Data from Walgreens.com. Drug information and prices. Available at: http://www.walgreens.com/pharmacy. Accessed December 1, 2003.

that must be taken seriously. Nurses must also be prepared to provide education for patients who are taking beta blockers and their families.

Metoprolol and bisoprolol may be administered without regard to food. However, they should be administered with or without food consistently to prevent variability of absorption. When administering beta blockers by the intravenous route, it is paramount to observe the specific recommendations for length of infusion. Metoprolol can be delivered undiluted at a rate of five milligrams per minute (ie, over 60 seconds). It is imperative to closely monitor blood pressure, heart rate, and electrocardiographic tracing during intravenous administration of metoprolol [25]. Carvedilol and bisoprolol are only available in oral form.

Nurses must also remember to obtain a baseline measure of heart rate and blood pressure before administering drugs and to report significant changes to the physician. Patients or families should be taught to monitor heart rate and blood pressure on a consistent basis. A target heart rate and blood pressure should be identified by the physician and documented so that

Table 3
Beta blocker therapy: contraindication

	Metoprolol	Carvedilol
Patients who have decompensated cardiac failure requiring intravenous inotropic therapy		X
Bronchial asthma or related bronch-spastic conditions		X
Second or third degree AV block, sick sinus syndrome, and severe bradycardia (except in patients who have a functioning pacemaker)		X
Cardiogenic shock	X	X
Severe hepatic failure	X	X
Pregnancy (2nd and 3rd trimesters)	X	X
Sinus bradycardia	X	
Heart block greater than first degree (except in patients who have a functioning artificial pacemaker)	X	
Uncompensated heart failure	X	

Data from Lacey CF, Armstrong LL, Goldman MP, et al. Drug information handbook. 10th edition. Ohio: Lexi-Comp; 2002.

nurses and patients will have guidelines for reporting. Bradycardia and hypotension may warrant dosage adjustment [25]. It is also important to advise patients to rise slowly, especially early in the up-titration process, because orthostatic hypotension may develop [26]. Dosing of beta blockers begins at very low doses and is up-titrated approximately every two weeks until the desired outcome is achieved or the maximum dose is reached [3]. Especially during this time of up-titration, patients should be monitored carefully for worsening of heart failure. Nurses should be consistently assessing these patients for dyspnea on exertion, orthopnea, and development of edema, shortness of breath, weight gain, wet lungs, and jugular venous distention. Patients who had chronic lung disease or asthma should be closely monitored for bronchospasm, especially with the administration of nonselective beta blockers [3].

Beta blocker therapy should never be discontinued abruptly, but should be withdrawn gradually to prevent adverse reactions such as anginal attacks, myocardial infarction, or worsening of heart failure. Blood pressure should be monitored frequently during withdrawal to detect rebound hypertension [25].

It is also important to remember that beta blockers may mask symptoms of hypoglycemia and hyperthyroidism. Diabetics must be closely monitored for decreased blood sugar and signs and symptoms of hypoglycemia that are not affected by beta blockers, such as diaphoresis, hunger, fatigue, mood changes, and inability to concentrate. Patients must be taught to be alert to these signs and symptoms and to perform self monitoring of blood glucose. Patients who have hyperthyroidism should have their thyroid levels monitored closely during beta blocker therapy. Abrupt withdrawal of beta blocker therapy may precipitate thyroid storm [25].

Consideration for drug withdrawal may be given if patients develop mental depression, because this can progress to catatonia. Patients should be observed closely for signs of depression, such as withdrawal, apathy, sadness, insomnia, difficulty concentrating, and disinterest in personal hygiene, dress, other people, and surroundings [25].

As symptom improvement may not occur for several months, it is important to make patients aware that continuation of the drug is important. Because fatigue may be prevalent during the first few weeks as a result of decreased sympathetic activity, patients may become discouraged and stop taking the medication [27].

Guidelines for administration

It is especially important that nurses be familiar with standard treatment of heart failure as it relates to beta blocker therapy. The Heart Failure Society of America has established guidelines for use in clinical practice. A summary of those guidelines as they relate to beta blocker therapy is outlined in Box 1. The three beta blocking medications recommended in

---

Box 1. Heart Failure Society of America practice guidelines for the management of heart failure: pharmacologic approaches and beta blocker therapy recommendations

- Administer beta blocker therapy to stable patients who have an ejection fraction of 40% or less and are NYHA Class II or III and are receiving standard therapy usually consisting of diuretics, ACE inhibitors, and digoxin.
- Consider beta blocker therapy for patients who are asymptomatic but have an ejection fraction of ≤40% and are currently undergoing standard therapy.
- Maintain standard therapy until patients are stable before initiating beta blocker therapy.
- Administer beta blocker therapy for patients who are symptomatic at rest.
- Initiate beta blocker therapy at low doses and up-titrate slowly at approximately 2-week intervals, performing clinical evaluations at each interval to detect worsening heart failure or other adverse reactions that may require dosage adjustment or termination.
- Continue beta blocker therapy in patients who experience exacerbation of symptoms during maintenance treatment.
- Provide proper patient education regarding early recognition of exacerbation and side effects.

Adapted from Heart Failure Society of America. Heart Failure Society of America (HSFA) Practice Guidelines: HSFA guidelines for management of patients with heart failure caused by left ventricular systolic dysfunction - pharmacologic approaches. Available at http://www.hfsa.org. Accessed December 1, 2003.

---

these guidelines are metoprolol, bisoprolol, and carvedilol [28]. The dosage titration that is recommended for treatment in heart failure is outlined in Table 4.

Summary

There is overwhelming evidence that beta blocker therapy in the form of metoprolol, bisoprolol, and carvedilol can have positive outcomes on morbidity, mortality, and quality of life in patients who have been diagnosed with mild to severe heart failure. Barring contraindications, beta blockers should be considered a cornerstone of therapy for these patients along with ACE inhibitors and diuretics. Beta blocking drugs are effective in modifying the cascade of events that occur as a result of the neurohormonal response that leads to the devastating effects evident during

Table 4
Initial and target doses for beta-blocker therapy in heart failure

Beta blocker	Starting dose	Target dose	Comments
Bisoprolol	1.25 mg/d	10 mg/d	β_1 selective: possible benefit in patients who have reactive airway disease Inconvenient dosage forms for initial titration
Carvedilol	3.125 mg/bid	25–50 mg/bid	FDA approved for treatment of HF Nonselective beta blocker/α_1 blocker Possible greater reduction in blood pressure (α_1 blocking effects) Convenient dosages
Metoprolol XL/CR	12.5–25 mg/d	200 mg/d	Compelling data for mortality benefit β_1 selective: possible benefit for patients who have reactive airway disease Inconvenient dosage forms for initial dose titration Less potential to decrease blood pressure (no α_1 blocking properties)

Abbreviation: FDA, Food and Drug Administration.
Data from Hunt SA, Baker DW, Chin MH et al. ACC/AHA guidelines for the evaluation and management of chronic heart failure in the adult: a report of the American College of Cardiology/American Heart Association Task Force on Practice Guidelines 2001. Available at http://www.acc.org/clinical/guidelines/failure/hf-index.htm. Accessed December 1, 2003; and Lacy CF, Armstrong LL, Goldman MP, Lance LL. *Drug Information Handbook.* 10th edition. Ohio: Lexi-Comp; 2002.

heart failure. Long-term effects of beta blockade include an increase in cardiac output, an increase in exercise tolerance, a decrease in the number of hospitalizations, and an overall improvement in symptoms [29].

References

[1] Hunt SA, Baker DW, Chin MH, et al. ACC/AHA guidelines for the evaluation and management of chronic heart failure in the adult: a report of the American College of Cardiology/American Heart Association Task Force on Practice Guidelines 2001. Available at: http://www.acc.org/clinical/guidelines/failure/hf_index.htm. Accessed December 1, 2003.

[2] Levy D, Kenchaiah S, Larson MG, et al. Long-term trends in the incidence of and survival with heart failure. N Engl J Med 2002;347(18):1397–444.

[3] Capriotti T. Current concepts and pharmacologic treatment of heart failure. Medsurg Nurs 2002;11(2):71–84.

[4] Futterman LG, Lemberg L. Heart failure: update on treatment and prognosis. Am J Crit Care 2001;10(4):285–93.

[5] Carelock J, Clark AP. Heart failure: pathophysiologic mechanisms. Am J Nurs 2001; 101(12):26–47.

[6] Pepper GS, Lee RW. Sympathetic activation in heart failure and its treatment with beta-blockade. Arch Intern Med 1999;159:225–34.

[7] Smith AL, Brown CS. New advances and novel treatments in heart failure. Crit Care Nurse 2003;23(Suppl):S11–20.

[8] Taccetta-Chapnick M. Using carvedilol to treat heart failure. Crit Care Nurse 2002;22(2): 36–58.

[9] Ignatavicius DD, Workman ML, Mishler MA. Medical-surgical nursing across the health care continuum. 3rd edition. Philadelphia: Saunders; 1999.

[10] Meghani SH, Becker D. Beta-blockers: a new therapy in congestive heart failure. Am J Crit Care 2001;10(6):417–28.

[11] Packer M, Coats A, Fowler MB, et al. Effect of carvedilol on survival in severe chronic heart failure. N Engl J Med 2001;344(22):1651–8.

[12] Skrabal MZ, Stading JA, Behmer-Miller KA, et al. Advances in the treatment of congestive heart failure: new approaches for an old disease. Pharmacotherapy 2000;20(7):787–804.

[13] Constant J. A review of why and how we may use beta-blockers in congestive heart failure. Chest 1998;113:800–8.

[14] Azevedo ER, Kubo T, Mak S, et al. Nonselective versus selective beta-adrenergic receptor blockade in congestive heart failure: differential effects on sympathetic activity. Circulation 2001;104(18):2194–200.

[15] The cardiac insufficiency bisoprolol study II (CIBIS-II): a randomised trial. Lancet 1999;353: 9–13.

[16] Effect of metoprolol CR/XL in chronic heart failure: Metoprolol CR/XL Randomised Intervention Trial in Congestive Heart Failure (MERIT-HF). Lancet 1999;353:2001–7.

[17] Gottlieb SS, Fisher ML, Kjekshus J, et al. Tolerability of beta-blocker initiation and titration in the Metoprolol CR/XL Randomized Intervention Trial in Congestive Heart Failure (MERIT-HF). Circulation 2002;105(10):1182–8.

[18] Poole-Wilson PA, Swedberg K, Cleland JG, et al. Comparison of carvedilol and metoprolol on clinical outcomes in patients with chronic heart failure in the Carvedilol Or Metoprolol European trial (COMET): randomised controlled trial. Lancet 2003;362(9377):7–13.

[19] Metra M, Giubbini R, Nodari S, et al. Differential effects of beta-blockers in patients with heart failure: a prospective, randomized, double-blind comparison of the long-term effects of metoprolol versus carvedilol. Circulation 2000;102:546–51.

[20] Eichhorn EJ, Domanski MJ, Krause-Steinrauf MS, et al. A trial of the beta-blocker bucindolol in patients with advanced chronic heart failure. N Engl J Med 2001;344(22): 1659–67.

[21] Lechat P, Packer M, Chalon S, et al. Clinical effects of B-adrenergic blockade in chronic heart failure: a meta-analysis of double-blind, placebo-controlled, randomized trials. Circulation 1998;98:1184–91.

[22] Krum H, Roecker EB, Mohacsi P, et al. Effects of initiating carvedilol in patients with severe chronic heart failure: results from the COPERNICUS study. JAMA 2003;289(6):712–8.

[23] Lacey CF, Armstrong LL, Goldman MP, et al. Drug information handbook. 10th edition. Ohio: Lexi-Comp; 2002.

[24] Walgreens.com. Drug information and prices Available at: http://www.walgreens.com/pharmacy. Accessed June, 2004.

[25] Wilson BA, Shannon MT, Stang CL. Nurse's drug guide 2001. New Jersey: Prentice Hall; 2000.

[26] New heart failure guidelines expand treatment options. RN 2003;66(4):26ac8–26ac10.

[27] Garg RK, Sorrentino MJ. Beta blockers for CHF. Adrenergic blockade dramatically reduces morbidity and mortality. Postgrad Med 2001;109(3):49–56.

[28] Heart Failure Society of America Heart Failure Society of America (HSFA) Practice Guidelines: HSFA guidelines for management of patients with heart failure caused by left ventricular systolic dysfunction – pharmacologic approaches. Available at: http://www.hfsa.org.

[29] Chavey WE II. The importance of beta blockers in the treatment of heart failure. Am Fam Physician 2000;62:2453–62.

ELSEVIER
SAUNDERS

NURSING
CLINICS
OF NORTH AMERICA

Nurs Clin N Am 40 (2005) 149–165

Update on Antiviral Agents for HIV and AIDS

Linda W. Covington, PhD, RN

School of Nursing, Middle Tennessee State University, Murfreesboro, TN 37132, USA

HIV primarily infects cells in the immune system. A protein on specific cells called CD4 allows HIV to enter and release viral RNA. The newly formed HIV virus then leaves the cell, destroying the CD4 cell in the process. When HIV enters the body, antibodies are created by the immune system to destroy the infected cells. Most treatments focus on eliminating infected cells and preventing proliferation of new HIV cells. Nurses caring for HIV patients must commit to continuous education, as HIV treatment regimens are constantly changing.

Case study

Mrs. G, a 40-year-old, middle-class mother of three was admitted to the hospital with fever, weight loss, productive cough, and diarrhea. Eight years earlier, Mrs. G gave birth to her third child by ceasarean section. She later developed postoperative hemorrhage and circulatory shock. Four units of blood were transfused. Several weeks after discharge, Mrs. G developed what she thought was the flu. After a week of rest, she recovered. Over the past 6 years, Mrs. G has gone to the physician with complaints of constant exhaustion and frequent colds. She was sent home and told to "take it easy." Over the past year, Mrs. G was hospitalized for a respiratory infection and what she thought was diarrhea from a stomach virus. In both cases, she was treated with medications and released. Mrs. G's condition continued to deteriorate. Most recently, Mrs. G was again brought to the hospital, where her husband insisted that the staff find out what was wrong with his wife. On assessment, she had a fever, tachypnea, severe diarrhea, and a productive cough. Her lymph nodes were enlarged and she had white patches in her mouth. After testing, it was determined that Mrs. G had

E-mail address: lcovingt@mtsu.edu

pneumocystic carinii pneumonia. Her admission diagnosis was AIDS. The reader may consider the following questions:

1. Why do you think Mrs. G's condition deteriorated without appropriate early intervention?
2. Would you have suspected that Mrs. G had AIDS?
3. Would you have known the appropriate treatment for Mrs. G?
4. Would you have known what laboratory tests to perform to monitor her progress?
5. What medication side effects would you expect?
6. Which drugs have the potential to interact?

   Unfortunately, there continues to be a lack of knowledge regarding treatments for patients diagnosed as having HIV or AIDS, especially among nurses who do not specialize in HIV care [1]. At a time when clients are entering hospitals sicker than ever, nurses must be aware of appropriate treatments either to cure diseases or promote a better quality of life. This is especially true for clients with depressed immune systems and, in particular, those who have HIV, which causes AIDS.

   Modes of transmission for HIV include sexual contact, blood contact, or in-utero transmission [2]. Although the virus has been transmitted to health care workers, this is uncommon. HIV infection is caused by a retrovirus that attacks the immune system. There are two types of HIV viruses: HIV-1, which is the primary cause of AIDS worldwide, and HIV-2, which is found mostly in West Africa [3,4]. This article focuses on HIV-1 occurring in the United States.

   In recent years, tremendous breakthroughs have occurred in the fight against HIV and AIDS. However, the struggle is far from over. The Centers for Disease Control and Prevention (CDC) estimates that 886,575 people in the United States have been diagnosed with AIDS since the beginning of the epidemic. The number of adults and adolescents with AIDS in the United States includes approximately 718,002 males and 159,271 females, with 9300 AIDS cases occurring in children younger than 13 years [3]. As of 2002, more than 350,000 people were living with AIDS. Since the start of the epidemic, approximately 501,669 people have died with AIDS, including 496,354 adults and adolescents and 5315 children younger than 15 years [3,5].

   The estimated number of new adult and adolescent HIV and AIDS cases in 2002 was 42,136, consisting of 70% men and 30% women. Of these newly infected people, half are younger than 25 years [2,6]. Subsequently, AIDS is now the fifth leading cause of death in the United States among people aged 25 to 44, and is the first leading cause of death for black men in this age group. Among black women in this age group, HIV ranks third [2,5]. Although the numbers are depressing, recent statistics are encouraging: it is estimated that AIDS-related deaths in the United States fell approximately 70% from 1995 to 1999, and from 51,117 deaths in 1995 to 16,371 deaths in 2002 [4,7].

Clients are often diagnosed as having HIV or AIDS after the immune system has already been destroyed. Consequently, these individuals are admitted to the hospital with a high acuity level and the intensive care nurse is often one of the first contacts within the health care system. Because nurses are responsible for treating clients with immunosuppression, they should be knowledgeable about appropriate drug therapy and its impact on the body.

Viral progression

A variety of cells have proteins on their surface that are called CD4 receptors. Although HIV infects a variety of cells, its main target is the T4 lymphocyte, a type of white blood cell that has numerous CD4 receptors. The T4 cell is responsible for warning the immune system that there are invaders in the system and is referred to as the master T cell. HIV searches for cells that have CD4 surface receptors, because this particular protein enables the virus to bind to the cell [8,9]. HIV mostly infects cells in the immune system. In addition to T lymphocytes (helper T cells), HIV recognizes and binds with CD4 molecules found on the outer surface of other cells, specifically monocytes, macrophages, and follicular dendrite cells in lymph nodes.

HIV is a retrovirus. Unlike other viruses, retroviruses have positive single-stranded RNA as their genetic material. To replicate, RNA is transformed into DNA by a process that involves the enzyme reverse transcriptase [10]. As the virus binds to the new blood cells, the blood cells produce new proteins which enable the viruses to stay alive and reproduce. Viruses hide their own DNA in the DNA of the infected cell so that when the cell produces new proteins, it also produces new viruses [8,9].

CD4 allows HIV to enter healthy cells and release viral RNA. Reverse transcriptase allows the single strand of RNA to convert to a double strand of complementary DNA (cDNA). A viral enzyme called integrase allows cDNA to copy into the host and replicate. Viruses released from the host require maturation to infect new cells. The HIV enzyme protease is required for this step, ensuring maturation and initiation of the infectious process [9]. Once the virus infects the CD4 cell, it seizes the genetic tools within the cell to manufacture new HIV virus. The newly formed HIV virus then leaves the cell, destroying the CD4 cell in the process.

The average healthy person has over 1000 CD4 cells/μL of blood. In a person infected with HIV, the virus mutates over time, presenting a slightly different arrangement with each generation while steadily destroying CD4 cells [10]. This destruction occurs over a period of years, diminishing the cells' protective ability and weakening the immune system. When the density of CD4 cells drops to 200 cells/μL of blood, the infected person becomes vulnerable to opportunistic infections and rare cancers [11].

Progression of HIV-1 infection to AIDS can occur within weeks or years. Usually within 1 to 3 weeks after primary infection with HIV most people experience flu-like symptoms, such as fever, muscle aches, sore throat, headache, skin rash, tender lymph nodes, and a vague feeling of discomfort that lasts 1 to 4 weeks. During this phase, called acute retroviral syndrome, HIV follows a triphasic clinical course in which massive replication causes a rapid rise of HIV in the blood [10]. The virus circulates throughout the body in the blood, particularly concentrating in organs of the lymphatic system. Even when there is an absence of symptoms, individuals infected with HIV are able to transmit the virus. The stage between initial exposure to the virus and before antibodies are detectable in the blood is known as the window period. The point at which HIV antibodies are present in the blood is called seroconversion [12]. Seroconversion usually occurs 1 to 3 months after exposure. During the next phase, a dramatic decline in the rate of viral replication occurs with an effective immune system. Individuals are usually asymptomatic because the virus disappears from the blood and reproduces in lymphoid tissue. A variety of symptoms that are debilitating, but not life-threatening, are experienced, such as weight loss and fatigue (ie, wasting syndrome), periodic fever, frequent diarrhea, and thrush, and recurring vaginal yeast in women [8,10]. When HIV infection reduces the number of CD4 cells to around 200 cells/μL of blood and the viral load increases to significant levels, the infected individual enters an early symptomatic phase known as latency, which lasts a few months to several years and may progress to AIDS [13,14]. Patients who are in this latency period develop opportunistic infections.

Diagnostic tests

Since 1983 when HIV was first identified as the cause of AIDS,various tests have been developed to help diagnose HIV infection and determine how far the infection has progressed. Other tests are used to screen donated blood, blood products, and body organs for the presence of HIV. Decisions regarding initiation or changes in antiretroviral therapy should be guided by the laboratory parameters of plasma HIV RNA (ie, viral load) measurements and CD4+ T cell counts [12].

Before deciding on therapy initiation, the CD4+ T lymphocyte count and plasma HIV RNA measurement should be performed twice to ensure accuracy and consistency, although antiretroviral therapy for patients who have advanced HIV should be initiated after the first viral load measurement is obtained to prevent a potentially harmful delay in treatment [7]. Plasma HIV RNA levels should not be measured during or within the 4 weeks after successful treatment of any infection, illness, or immunization. Because there are differences in the confirmatory tests, HIV RNA levels should be measured by the same laboratory and technique to ensure accuracy.

Presence of the virus in the body is determined by identifying HIV antibodies, which are specialized proteins created by the immune system to destroy the virus [14]. HIV antibodies develop anywhere from 5 weeks to 3 months after HIV infection occurs, depending on the individual's immune system. The antibodies are produced continually throughout the course of the infection [8–10].

The standard test to detect HIV antibodies in the blood is the ELISA. In this test, a blood sample is mixed with proteins from HIV. If the blood contains HIV antibodies, they attach to the HIV proteins, producing a color change in the mixture. This test is highly reliable when performed 2 to 3 months after infection, but less reliable when used in the very early stage of infection, before detectable levels of antibodies have had a chance to build [12].

Western blot analysis or an immunofluorescence assay should be used to confirm a positive ELISA. Western blotting can detect lower levels of HIV antibodies. The combination of the ELISA and Western blot assays detects HIV infection with 99.9% accuracy within 12 weeks following exposure. A modified ELISA test that detects p24 antigen, which is a protein produced by the virus, can determine if specific drug treatments are having a positive effect on a patient who has HIV.

Other techniques used to determine HIV presence and duration of infection include: (1) the Detuned test, which is used after Western blotting to determine if the HIV infection occurred within last 6 months [12]; (2) oral mucosal transudate-based testing, which is a new method that detects antibodies in the oral fluids [12]; and (3) urine testing, which is used only to detect viral antibodies, not HIV particles, because urine does not contain the virus [12].

CD4 cell counts

Once tests confirm an HIV infection, CD4 blood levels should be periodically monitored. The progressive loss of CD4 cells corresponds to a worsening of the disease as the immune system becomes increasingly impaired. Cell counts should be measured at the time of diagnosis and every 3 to 6 months thereafter. CD4 count and percentages reflect immune status, not HIV activity [12].

The CD4 count is calculated based on the percentage of CD4 cells present in the total lymphocyte count:

- Normal count is 800 to 1100 cells/mm^3 or 40% of total.
- <500 cells/mm^3 is considered low.
- <200 cells/mm^3 is criterion for diagnosing AIDS.

Pagana K, Pagana T. Mosby's manual of diagnostic and laboratory tests. St. Louis, MO: Mosby; 2002.

A decrease in CD4+ T-lymphocyte count is considered substantial when it is more than 30% from baseline for absolute cell numbers, and more than 3% from baseline in percentages of cells [7,12].

Viral load

Viral load tests measure the amount of the virus in the blood using polymerase chain reaction (PCR) technology. PCR tests measure the level of viral RNA in blood to determine the rate of HIV growth in an infected person. The result of a viral load test is described as the number of copies of HIV RNA per milliliter (copies/mL). Ten thousand or fewer copies/mL is generally considered low, and 50,000 or more copies/mL is considered high [2,9,12].

Awareness of the viral load helps in estimating survival time. For example, studies show that without treatment, the average survival time for people with an HIV viral load more than 30,000 per microliter of blood is 4.4 years, while those with a viral load less than 10,000 cells/μL of blood live for an average of 10 years. The Food and Drug Administration (FDA) has approved three HIV viral load assays for use in determining prognosis and response to therapy. These include: (1) the HIV-1 reverse transcriptase polymerase chain reaction assay, (2) the in vitro nucleic amplification test for HIV-RNA, and (3) the in vitro signal–amplification nucleic acid probe assay.

Undetectable viral loads are described as 50 copies/mL or fewer when tested using the PCR assay. This does not mean that there is no HIV in the sample, just that the number of copies is somewhere between 0 and 49 [3,12]. In vitro nucleic amplification and in vitro signal–amplification nucleic acid probe assays were approved for a lower limit of detection at 50 copies/mL. Viral load testing is an essential parameter in deciding to initiate or change antiretroviral therapies. For the untreated patient, viral load testing using quantitative methods should be performed at the time of diagnosis and every 3 to 4 months thereafter [15]. The more HIV present in the blood, the faster CD4 T cells (ie, essential immune system cells that fight infection) are lost [14], thereby increasing the risk that symptoms will manifest in the next few years [15].

Viral load levels should also be measured immediately before initiation of antiretroviral therapy and 2 to 8 weeks thereafter to determine therapy effectiveness. According to CDC guidelines, adherence to a regimen of potent antiretroviral agents should result in a substantial decrease (approximately 1.0 log10) in viral load by 2 to 8 weeks. The viral load should continue to decline over the following weeks and, for the majority of patients, should decrease below detectable levels. With optimal therapy, viral levels in plasma at 24 weeks should be below the limit of detection [12–14].

Goals of therapy

Where it has succeeded, antiviral therapy has transformed an almost fatal illness into a manageable chronic condition. Antiviral drugs inhibit viral replication, but do not eliminate viruses from tissues. Antiviral therapy is usually recommended for patients who have CD4 cell counts that are less than 500, viral loads of 20,000 copies of HIV RNA per milliliter of plasma, or more than 10,000 (bDNA) [10]. Therapy is aimed at:

- Suppressing viral replication
- Reducing viral loads to undetectable levels
- Improving the quality of life
- Prolonging health by enhancing the immune system
- Decreasing the risk of drug resistance
- Reducing HIV-related morbidity and mortality

Treatment of HIV and AIDS has been difficult because of the length of time the virus remains dormant in the T cells and because of the side effects of the drugs. Once a patient begins antiviral therapy, the drugs must be taken as prescribed. When a drug is stopped, it cannot be restarted because of the high risk of drug resistance. Therefore, before therapy is initiated, patients must be prepared to make a lifelong commitment to regimen adherence, and possible toxicities must be considered [13].

Although drastic improvements have been made in the fight against HIV and AIDS as a result of highly active antiretroviral therapy (HAART), antiviral drugs remain limited and difficult to develop [14]. As of December 2003, approximately 20 different drugs are available for treatment of HIV and AIDS. Most of the recent research has supported the concurrent use of two or three drugs to completely suppress the virus. For example, the combination of zidovudine, lamivudine, and efavirenz has been an effective initial treatment. This combination appears to suppress the virus more quickly and for a longer period of time [16].

Antiviral therapy

The HIV enzyme integrase helps the newly formed viral DNA become part of the structure of the infected cell's DNA. The viral DNA then forces the infected cell to manufacture HIV particles. Another HIV enzyme, protease, then packages these HIV particles into a complete and functional HIV virus. A variety of drugs that block enzyme actions in HIV replication have been developed over the past 15 years. There are currently four major classes of antiretroviral drugs in general use: (1) nucleoside analog reverse transcriptase inhibitors (NRTIs), (2) nonnucleoside reverse transcriptase inhibitors (NNRTIs), (3) protease inhibitors (PIs), and (4) fusion inhibitors [2,9,11,13].

Nucleoside reverse transcriptase inhibitors

NRTIs, also called <u>nucleoside analogs</u>, are similar to the natural building blocks of DNA in their purine nucleosides adenosine and guanosine, and their pyrimidine nucleosides thymidine and cytidine. Consequently, they easily enter the DNA of viruses present in cells. NRTIs function by impeding the action of the viral enzyme reverse transcriptase, which converts the virus's genetic material into DNA. This action inhibits reverse transcriptase from synthesizing DNA, thus preventing viral enzymes from being replicated in the newly infected cell. These drugs incorporate themselves into the structure of the viral DNA, rendering the DNA useless [2,11,14].

NRTIs are triphosphorylated intracellularly to become nucleotides. Their presence in the DNA halts transcription. Unfortunately, these drugs can also function as substrates for other enzymes capable of DNA formation, including human DNA polymerase and b gamma, the only enzyme involved in the replication of mitochondrial DNA. Mitochondrial function can be disrupted through NRTI-mediated inhibition of this enzyme [17]. Regrettably, most patients experience side effects after prolong use. The toxic effects of NRTIs are related to mitochondrial damage. Adverse events from this inhibition can lead to fatal lactic acidosis. Other serious complications include fat loss in the extremities and hepatotoxicity.

The nucleoside analog known as azidothymidine (AZT) became available in 1987 and was the first drug approved by the United States Food and Drug Administration (FDA) to treat AIDS. AZT slows HIV proliferation in the body by permitting an increase in the number of CD4 cells, thereby boosting the immune system. AZT also prevents transmission of HIV from an infected mother to her newborn. Since the introduction of AZT, additional nucleoside analogs have been developed, including didanosine (Videx), zalcitabine (HIVID), stavudine (Zerit), lamivudine (Epivir), and abacavir (Ziagen) Table 1. These drugs are not particularly powerful when used alone—often their benefits last for only 6 to 12 months. But when nucleoside analogs are used in combination with each other, they provide longer-lasting and more effective results. This group of drugs is typically included in the front-line treatment of HIV and known as HAART [2,8–11,13].

Nucleotide reverse transcriptase inhibitors, or nucleotide analogs, resemble monophosphorylated nucleosides, and therefore require only two additional phosphorylations to become active inhibitors of DNA synthesis Table 2. Reverse transcriptase fails to distinguish the phosphorylated NRTIs from their natural counterparts and attempts to use the drugs in the synthesis of viral DNA. When an NRTI is incorporated into a strand of DNA being synthesized, the addition of further nucleotides is prevented and a full-length copy of the viral DNA is not produced [2,9–11,13].

Table 1
Characteristics of nucleoside reverse transcriptase inhibitors

Generic (trade name)	Adverse effects	Dosages
Zidovudine (AZT, ZDV, Retrovir) Primary drug of choice in asymptomatic and advanced HIV; absorbed orally, metabolized in liver	Bone marrow suppression, severe anemia, neutropenia, granulocytopenia, neurotoxicity (CNS: anxiety, headache, irritability, sleeplessness), peripheral neuropathy, fat redistribution, acidosis, liver failure. gastrointestinal intolerance, insomnia, lactic acidosis with hepatic steatosis (rare but potentially life-threatening toxicity associated with using NRTIs).	Asymptomatic HIV: 100 mg q 4 hr (total 500 mg); when given in combination, the dosage may be extended to q 8 hr Symptomatic HIV- 100 mg q 4 hr (total 600 mg) 300 mg bid or 200 mg tid
Abacavir (Ziagen) Used only in combination therapy. Take without regard to meals. Alcohol increases drug levels. Absorbed orally.	Hypersensitivity reaction (which can be fatal) is an absolute contraindication for reusing this drug. Symptoms may include fever, rash, nausea, vomiting, malaise or fatigue, loss of appetite, respiratory symptoms such as sore throat, cough, shortness of breath	300 mg bid or with ZDV and 3TC as Trizivir, 1 dose bid
Didanosine (ddI, Videx) Take 1/2 h before or 2 h after meals; given when unable to tolerate Zidovudine.	Has poor bioavailability— destroyed by stomach acid. Pancreatitis, nausea, diarrhea, lactic acidosis with hepatic steatosis is a rare but potentially life-threatening toxicity, peripheral neuropathy (rare)	Body weight $\geq$ 60 kg 400 mg qd (buffered tablets or enteric coated capsule), or 200 mg bid (buffered tablets); body weight <60 kg: 250 mg qd (buffered tablets or enteric coated capsule), or 125 mg bid (buffered tablets)
Lamivudine (Epivir) Used in advanced HIV with ZDV or other drugs to slow the resistance development	Rare side effects: pancreatitis (with abdominal pain, nausea, vomiting), lactic acidosis with hepatic steatosis	Body weight <50 kg: 150 mg bid, or 300 mg qd with ZDV; dose is reduced with renal damage
Stavudine (Zerit) Take without regard to meals; used in advanced HIV if other HIV drugs are not tolerated	Peripheral neuropathy, lipodystrophy, rapidly progressive ascending neuromuscular weakness (rare), pancreatitis, lactic acidosis with hepatic steatosis	$\geq$60 kg 40 mg PO q 12 h <60 kg 30 mg PO q 12 h
Zalcitabine (Hivid) Take without regard to meals; used with Zidovudine to treat advanced HIV	Peripheral neuropathy	0.75 mg q 8 h tid (2.25 mg/d)

Table 1 *(continued)*

Generic (trade name)	Adverse effects	Dosages
Emtricitabine (Emtriva) (take without regard to meals)	Minimal toxicity, lactic acidosis with hepatic steatosis, headache, diarrhea, lack of appetite, fatigue	200 mg capsule once a day

Abbreviations: CNS, central nervous system; NRTI, nucleoside reverse transcriptase inhibitor.

Data from Refs. [2,9,11,13].

Table 2
Characteristics of nucleotide reverse transcriptase inhibitors

Generic (trade name)	Adverse effects	Dosage and food effects
Tenofovir, Tenofovir disoproxil fumarate (Viread, PMPA)	Diarrhea, flatulence, nausea, vomiting, possible bone damage (only confirmed in animals), asthenia, headache, rare reports of renal insufficiency; contraindicated in pregnancy; if combined with didanosine, can increase drug levels and increase risk of fatal pancreatitis	Take 300 mg qd without regard to meals; administered orally, absorbed best with food; fats increase absorption

From Aidsinfo. A service of the US Department of Health and Human Services. Available at: http://www.aidsinfo.nih.gov/drugs/. Accessed February 24, 2004.

Non-nucleoside reverse transcriptase inhibitors

NNRTIs were introduced in 1996. This group of drugs prevents the enzyme activity that converts RNA to DNA, thereby inhibiting viral replication. These drugs bind directly to block reverse transcriptase. Three NNRTIs are available: nevirapine (Viramune), delavirdine (Rescriptor), and efavirenz (Sustiva) Table 3. NNRTIs work best when used in combination with nucleoside analogs [2,9,11,13].

Protease inhibitors

The third group of antiviral drugs, protease inhibitors (PIs), attack HIV-infected cells by inhibiting the protease enzymes that are required for maturation of cells. When these drugs block protease, defective HIV particles form that are unable to infect new cells. PIs bind to the active site of the viral protease enzyme, preventing viral proteins from being processed into functional forms. When this binding occurs, immature cells are formed that are not capable of replication. Viral particles are still produced when protease is inhibited, but these particles are ineffective at infecting new cells. Two major concerns with the use of PIs are drug resistance and interaction. Approximately half of the patients develop resistance within the first year of therapy.

Table 3
Characteristics of non-nucleoside reverse transcriptase inhibitors

Generic (trade name)	Adverse effects	Dosage and food effects
Delavirdine (Rescriptor) Oral administration, used with NRTIs and protease inhibitors	Rash, increased transaminase levels, headaches	Take without regard to meals; 400 mg PO tid; four 100 mg tablets can be dispersed in ≥ 3 oz of water; 200 mg tablets should be taken as intact tablets; separate dosing with didanosine or antacids by 1 hour
Efavirenz (Sustiva)	Linked to CNS effects: bizarre dreams, dizziness, sleep disorders, aggression, depression, paranoia, suicidal thoughts ($<2\%$), increased transaminase levels; rash	600 mg PO daily on an empty stomach, preferably at bedtime; high-fat/high-caloric meals increase peak plasma concentrations
Nevirapine (Viramune)	Fatal hepatotoxicity, hepatitis, fatal skin reaction including Stevens-Johnson syndrome	Take without regard to meals; 200 mg PO qd for 14 d; thereafter, 200 mg PO bid

Abbreviations: NRTI, nucleoside reverse transcriptase inhibitor; CNS, central nervous system.

From Aidsinfo. A service of the US Department of Health and Human Services. Available at: http://www.aidsinfo.nih.gov/drugs/. Accessed February 2004.

PIs are more powerful than NRTIs and NNRTIs. These antiviral drugs produce dramatic decreases in HIV levels in the blood, which enables CD4 cell levels to drastically increase. The first PI saquinavir (Invirase) was approved in 1995. Since then other PIs have been approved, including ritonavir (Norvir), indinavir (Crixivan), nelfinavir (Viracept), and amprenavir (Agenerase) Table 4 [2,9–11,13].

Table 4
Characteristics of protease inhibitors

Generic (trade name)	Food effects	Adverse effects
Indinavir (Crixivan)	Take 1 h before or 2 h after meals; or may take with skim milk or low-fat meal	Nephrolithiasis, GI intolerance, nausea, increased indirect bilirubinemia, headache, asthenia, blurred vision, dizziness, rash, metallic taste, thrombocytopenia, alopecia, hemolytic anemia, hyperglycemia, fat redistribution and lipid abnormalities, possible increased bleeding episodes[a]

Table 4 *(continued)*

Generic (trade name)	Food effects	Adverse effects
Amprenavir (Agenerase)	Can take with or without food, but high-fat meal should be avoided	GI intolerance, nausea, vomiting, diarrhea, rash, oral paresthesias, transaminase elevation, hyperglycemia, fat redistribution and lipid abnormalities, possible increased bleeding episodes[a]
Atazanavir (Reyataz)	Administer with food to increase bioavailability, does not appear to have harmful effects on cholesterol levels	Indirect hyperbilirubinemia, prolonged PR interval (may cause asymptomatic first degree AV block, use caution in patients with conduction defects or on other medications that cause PR prolongation), hyperglycemia, fat maldistribution, possible increased bleeding episodes[a], nausea, infection, headache, vomiting, diarrhea, abdominal pain, somnolence, insomnia, fever
Lopinavir + Ritonavir (Kaletra)	Take with food	GI intolerance, nausea, vomiting, diarrhea, asthenia, elevated transaminase enzymes, hyperglycemia, fat redistribution and lipid abnormalities, possible increased bleeding episodes[a], increases in cholesterol and triglycerides, increased liver enzymes (liver toxicity; oral solution contains 42% alcohol)
Nelfinavir (Viracept)	Take with meal or snack	Diarrhea, hyperglycemia, fat redistribution and lipid abnormalities, possible increased bleeding episodes[a], transaminase elevation
Ritonavir (Norvir)	Take with food if possible; this may improve tolerability	GI intolerance, nausea, vomiting, diarrhea, paresthesias, hepatitis, pancreatitis; asthenia, taste perversion, triglycerides increase >200%, transaminase elevation, elevated CPK and uric acid, hyperglycemia, fat redistribution and lipid abnormalities, possible increased bleeding episodes[a]

Table 4 *(continued)*

Generic (trade name)	Food effects	Adverse effects
Saquinavir (Invirase) (hard gel capsule)	No food effect when taken with ritonavir	GI intolerance, nausea and diarrhea, headache, elevated transaminase enzymes, hyperglycemia, fat redistribution and lipid abnormalities, possible increased bleeding episodes[a]
Saquinavir (Fortovase) (soft gel capsule)	Take with large meal	GI intolerance, nausea, diarrhea, abdominal pain and dyspepsia, headache; elevated transaminase enzymes, hyperglycemia, fat redistribution and lipid abnormalities, possible increased bleeding episodes[a]

Abbreviations: GI, gastrointestinal; AV, atrioventricular; CPK, creatine phosphokinase.
[a] in patients with hemophilia.

Fusion inhibitors

A new class of drugs called fusion inhibitors became available in 2003 when the FDA approved the use of enfuvirtide (Fuzeon) Table 5. Fusion inhibitors prevent HIV from entering target cells and binding to CD4 cells. Drugs of this class bind to the HIV envelope protein gp41, which is involved in viral entry. By blocking the interactions between regions of the gp41 protein, fusion inhibitors interfere with the conformational change of the envelope molecule required for fusion with the target cell membrane. When used with other antiretroviral medicines, fusion inhibitors can reduce the amount of HIV in the blood and increase the number of CD4 cells [2].

The diagnosis and treatment of patients who have HIV or AIDS is very challenging and constantly evolving. In addition to the tremendous physical alterations, these individuals have significant nutritional, psychosocial, and spiritual needs. Nurses fulfill a variety of roles in screening, treating, educating, and supporting these individuals. Boxes 1 and 2 provide additional recommendations for nursing care of this complex population.

Table 5
Characteristics of fusion inhibitors

Generic (trade name)	Dosage	Adverse effects
Enfuvirtide (Fuzeon)	Injectable; in lyophilized powder 90 mg (1 mL) subcutaneously bid; each vial contains 108 mg to be reconstituted with 1.1 mL of sterile water	Local injection site reactions, increased rate of bacterial pneumonia, hypersensitivity reactions (<1%)

Box 1. Recommendations from the Panel of Clinical Practices for treatment of HIV infections

- Measure HIV RNA levels before starting therapy and repeat test 2 to 8 weeks after initiation. (The HIV RNA test is used to evaluate when to start therapy, regimen adherence, and response to therapy. This test measures HIV levels in the blood, but not in the tissues where replication may be continuing.)
- Initiate treatment for clients within 6 months of seroconversion, usually for a CD4+ count < 500 or a viral load > 10,000 plasma HIV RNA levels or 20,000 copies/mL.
- Use combination antiviral therapy if available, except during pregnancy.
- Typically, initiate three-drug regimen: two NRTIs and a protease inhibitor, two NRTIs and enfavirenz, or two protease inhibitors and one or two NRTIs. Side effects, health status, and ability to follow regimen should be considered when determining therapy.
- Start ritonavir and nevirapine at lower dosages and increase gradually. Start other drugs at therapeutic dose.
- Assess for adverse drug effects at least twice during the first month of treatment and every 3 months thereafter.
- Evaluate drug effectiveness: a reduction in HIV RNA levels should be noted by 2 months and levels should be nearly undetectable by 4 to 6 months. If these goals are not met, drug resistance, inadequate dosage, and nonadherence should be assessed.
- Refrain from interrupting drug therapy. Stopping therapy increases drug resistance.
- Continue medications during infections and malignancy, if possible.
- CD4+ cell count should be measured at the time of diagnosis and every 3 to 6 months afterward. The count should increase with effective treatment.

References [2,5,6,11,13].

Therapy and altered nutrition

Protein energy malnutrition in patients with HIV and AIDS has been a very common complication. Patients who experience weight loss and wasting are at higher risk for complications and opportunistic infections. Life expectancy and quality of life is expected to improve if the wasting

---

Box 2. Nursing care for the client with HIV or AIDS

Nursing assessment
- Assess baseline data to monitor response to therapy.
- Determine vital signs, weight, and nutritional status.
- Order laboratory tests (ie, CD4, viral load, CBC, renal and liver functions).

Nursing diagnoses
- Social isolation as a result of stigma associated with medical diagnosis.
- Altered body image caused by physiologic and psychosocial changes.
- Alteration in nutrition as a result of malabsorption or wasting syndrome.
- At risk for sensory deficit and injury resulting from problems such as weakness, infection, and drug reaction.
- Altered respiratory status as a result of fluid consolidation.
- Self-care difficulties related to weakness or systemic infection.
- Knowledge deficit regarding disease process or medication.

Planning
- Provide emotional support and counseling.
- Make sure drugs are not contraindicated before administering.
- Administer drugs as ordered; consider food effects, elimination pattern, and drug interactions.

Evaluation
- CDC-recommended guidelines for administration of antiviral drugs are followed by health care providers.
- Viral regression occurs with effective antiviral drugs.
- Patients exhibit increased CD4 levels and decreased viral load.

---

process can be reversed. However, this reversal has proven to be difficult. Findings suggest that increases in body weight have mainly been in the form of fat and water, rather than lean body mass. With the introduction of new antiretroviral agents, nutritional status and survival have improved, but metabolic abnormalities, such as lipodystrophy and metabolic syndrome (eg, Syndrome X), have also been prevalent.

Hypermetabolism is thought to play an integral role in weight loss and malnutrition in patients who have HIV or AIDS. Many studies found that resting energy expenditure (REE) was increased in patients with AIDS, especially in those who had secondary infections. Not all patients are hypermetabolic; some may even be hypometabolic (ie, have decreased REE). Hypometabolism is thought to be related to malabsorption. Alterations in lipid metabolism are also common in HIV infection. Increases in plasma-fasting triglyceride concentrations often occur, especially after HAART therapy is initiated. PI therapy has been shown to cause an increase in total cholesterol (eg, LDL and VLDL, but not HDL).

Abnormalities in glucose metabolism also occur in HIV patients. Patients who have advanced HIV have demonstrated significant increases in insulin clearance and sensitivity. The alterations in lipid and glucose metabolism may lead to increased risk of coronary disease in these patients. As a result of patients living longer, illnesses attributed to therapy or the disease itself are being experienced that were not previously observed, such as metabolic syndrome and increased risk of mortality related to coronary artery disease [18].

Summary

Drug therapy is a vital component of the care required to promote quality of life for individuals who are afflicted with HIV or AIDS. Issues including weight loss and gain, heart disease, insulin resistance, and even increased bone metabolism must be considered when determining appropriate pharmacologic therapy. New complications often arise with new treatments; living longer may not always mean living better. However, it is the responsibility of nurses to promote the best care possible. Management of appropriate drug therapy and the related implications are critical nursing responsibilities in the care of individuals who have HIV or AIDS.

References

[1] Hall J, Sutton A. Non-HIV nurses' knowledge of HIV therapy. Nurs Stand 2002;16(43): 33–6.

[2] Aidsinfo. A service of the US Department of Health and Human Services. Available at: http://www.aidsinfo.nih.gov/drugs/. Accessed February 24, 2004.

[3] Centers for Disease Control and Prevention. HIV prevention strategic plan through 2005. Available at: http://www.cdc.gov/hiv/stats.htm. Accessed February 18, 2004.

[4] Department of Human Services. National vital statistics reports. Hyattsville, MD: National Center for Health Statistics; 2001. Divisions of HIV/AIDS Prevention, Vol. 49, No. 8.

[5] Center for Disease Control. Cases of HIV infection and AIDS in the United States. Division of Statistics; 2002. HIV/AIDS surveillance report, Vol. 14. Atlanto (GA): Centers for Disease Control & Prevention.

[6] Fleming PL, Byers RH, Sweeney PA, et al. HIV prevalence in the United States, 2000. Presented at the 9th Annual Conference on Retroviruses and Opportunistic Infections. Seattle, February 24–28, 2002.

[7] Centers for Disease Control and Prevention. Cases of HIV infection and AIDS in the United States, 2002. Available at: http://www.cdc.gov/hiv/stats/hasr1402/table1.htm. Accessed February 20, 2004.

[8] Porth C. Pathophysiology: concepts of altered health states. 6th edition. Philadelphia: Lippincott; 2002.

[9] McKenry L, Salerno E. Pharmacology in nursing. 21st edition. St. Louis, MO: Mosby; 2003.

[10] Lehne R. Pharmacology for nursing care. 4th edition. Philadelphia: Saunders; 2001.

[11] Karch A. Focus on nursing pharmacology. 2nd edition. Philadelphia: Lippincott; 2003.
[12] Pagana K, Pagana T. Mosby's manual of diagnostic and laboratory tests. St. Louis, MO: Mosby; 2002.
[13] Queener S, Gutierrez K. Pharmacology for nursing practice. St. Louis, MO: Mosby; 2003.
[14] Abrams A. Clinical drug therapy: rationale for nursing practice. 6th edition. Philadelphia: Lippincott; 2003.
[15] Aidsmap treatment and care: viral load, CDC count and other tests. Available at: http://www.aidsmap.com. Accessed March 3, 2004.
[16] Robbins S. HIV therapy. N Engl J Med 2003;349:2351.
[17] Lonergan T, Barber E, Mathews C. Safety and efficacy of switching to alternative nucleoside analogues following symptomatic hyperlactatemia and lactic acidosis. AIDS 2003;17(17): 2495–9.
[18] Salas-Salvado J, Garcia-Lorda P. The metabolic puzzle during the evolution of HIV infection. Clin Nutr 2001;20:379–91.

ELSEVIER
SAUNDERS

Nurs Clin N Am 40 (2005) 167–182

NURSING
CLINICS
OF NORTH AMERICA

An Evaluation of Children's Metered-dose Inhaler Technique for Asthma Medications

Patricia V. Burkhart, PhD, RN[a],*,
Mary Kay Rayens, PhD[b],
Roxanne K. Bowman, BSN, RN[c]

[a]College of Nursing, Room 517, University of Kentucky, Lexington, KY 40536, USA
[b]Colleges of Nursing and Medicine, Room 543, University of Kentucky,
Lexington, KY 40536, USA
[c]Pediatric Nurse Practitioner Program, College of Nursing, Room 517,
University of Kentucky, Lexington, KY 40536, USA

Asthma is a chronic inflammatory disease of the airways that causes recurrent episodes of wheezing, coughing, shortness of breath, and chest tightness. There are more than 20 million Americans who have asthma, and 6.3 million of them are children [1]. Despite increased understanding of the pathogenesis of asthma and a number of efficacious therapies, asthma-associated morbidity in children is on the rise [1]. In 2000, asthma claimed the lives of 4487 people, including 223 children between infancy and 17 years of age [2].

Inhaled medications are the mainstay of asthma management and are generally delivered by a metered-dose inhaler (MDI). Improper MDI technique can result in decreased drug delivery to the distal airways and poor asthma outcomes. Inadequate asthma control may lead to an increase in acute care and hospital visits, a greater number of missed school days, and even death [3]. Improving drug delivery through proper technique is a simple, yet effective way to increase children's asthma symptom control.

This study was approved by the Medical Institutional Review Board at the University of Pittsburgh. Only children whose parents gave written consent for them to participate in the 5-week asthma self-management clinical trial were included.
 * Corresponding author.
 E-mail address: pvburk2@uky.edu (P.V. Burkhart).

Purpose

The purposes of this study were to: (1) describe the accuracy of children's MDI technique, (2) identify common mistakes made by children using MDIs, and (3) determine whether teaching the correct MDI technique to children resulted in fewer errors and improved performance. In addition, new drug delivery devices for asthma medications and their implications for patient care are discussed.

Review of relevant literature

The National Heart, Lung, and Blood Institute's [3] "Guidelines for the Diagnosis and Management of Asthma" identified pharmacologic therapy as integral to asthma management. Inhaled medications are frequently prescribed for children with asthma because they deliver the medication directly to the lungs, provide a faster onset of action, and allow smaller doses of the drug to be effective [4].

Unfortunately, many children who have asthma do not use their inhalers correctly. Scarfone et al [5] found that 45% of pediatric patients using an MDI (n = 73) and 44% using an MDI with a spacer (n = 135) during an acute asthma episode exhibited multiple errors in technique. Similarly, a review of 20 articles on MDI technique for both children and adults indicated the average incidence of inaccurate technique was 38% [6]. The principal errors were: (1) failure to coordinate actuation of the MDI with inhalation (27%), (2) holding the breath for too short a period after inhalation (26%), (3) inappropriate, rapid inspiration of the medication (19%), and (4) inadequate shaking of the medication before use (13%).

The problem of coordinating actuation with inhalation may be alleviated by the use of a holding chamber (ie, spacer). Holding chambers have a one-way valve that decreases the need for hand–breath coordination, thereby allowing more time for the patient to inhale the medication. Spacer devices improve drug deposition to the distal airways by allowing the larger particles to settle out and the smaller particles to deposit deeper in the lungs, rather than in the back of the throat [7]. With the exception of the breath-actuated MDI, a holding chamber is recommended for use with MDIs at all ages to improve technique [4,8]. MDIs with a spacer are as effective as nebulizers in delivering medication to children and are more cost-effective [9].

Assessing children's MDI technique at each health care encounter and teaching and reviewing children's medication administration technique, are critical to ensuring efficacy of the medication and improving asthma outcomes. The development of new inhaled medication devices presents challenges for health care providers and patients, requiring them to learn new administration techniques.

Methods

Design

MDI administration technique was assessed for children with persistent asthma who participated in a randomized, controlled intervention study evaluating the effectiveness of an asthma self-management program [10,11]. Pre- and postintervention assessments of the children's MDI technique were collected during two nurse-led asthma education sessions in the 5-week clinical trial. Teaching of appropriate MDI administration technique occurred after the baseline assessment and was reinforced after the postintervention assessment 1 to 4 weeks later.

Sample

A sample of children (N = 42) aged 7 through 11 years with persistent asthma was gathered from pediatric practices and public recruitment in West Virginia. Thirty-six of the 42 children remembered to bring their inhaled medications with dispensers and spacers (if used) to at least two of the asthma-education sessions. The six children who did not remember to bring their medications to at least two of the three sessions were not included in the assessment of MDI technique. The preintervention evaluation for MDI technique occurred either Week 1 or 2, and the postevaluation occurred 1 to 4 weeks later (Weeks 2 to 5), depending on when the children remembered to bring their medications. Seventy-two percent of the children were assessed 3 weeks apart, whereas 20% had assessments 1 week apart, and 8% were evaluated 4 weeks apart.

The mean age of the children was 9.6 years (SD = 1.6), with an age range of 7 through 11 years. As displayed in Table 1, the children were predominantly male, Caucasian (reflective of the rural area [3.3% minority] where the sample was recruited), and typically came from two-parent, middle- to high-income families. At the time of the study, the children were an average of 4.7 years (SD = 2.8) beyond their asthma diagnosis. Most of the children had never been hospitalized for asthma and reported having asthma symptoms weekly or monthly. The majority of parents stated that their child's asthma symptoms were under good to very good control. Asthma medication had been prescribed for all of the children.

Measures

The same nurse who was present at the asthma self-management sessions observed the MDI techniques and recorded on a checklist whether or not each of the correct steps for proper technique occurred. The six behavioral criteria used to determine accurate MDI technique included five from a measurement tool developed for a previous study [12]. A sixth criterion,

Table 1
Demographic and asthma characteristics of the sample (N = 36)

Characteristic	n	%
Gender		
Male	26	72
Female	10	28
Race		
Caucasian	35	97
Minority	1	3
Child lives with:		
Two parents	32	89
One parent	4	11
Health insurance		
Private	33	92
Assistance or no insurance	3	8
Number of asthma hospitalizations		
0	22	61
1 or more	14	39
Asthma symptom frequency		
Daily	9	25
Weekly or monthly	27	75
Parents' assessment of asthma control		
Very good/good	19	53
Fair/poor	17	47

the use of a spacer, was added to the assessment. The six criteria indicating correct technique were as follows:

- Canister was shaken before use.
- Good coordination present between activation and inspiration.
- Inhalation occurred to total lung capacity.
- Breath was held between two actuations.
- Canister was shaken before second actuation.
- Spacer was used (if appropriate for type of inhaler).

In addition to observing whether each of these correct behaviors occurred, the observer used a 3-point scale recommended by Hughes et al [12] to rate the child's MDI technique as "good," "fair," or "poor." Good MDI technique indicated that all of the behaviors were present, fair indicated that only some of the behaviors were present, and poor indicated that none of the behaviors was present.

Procedure

Children's technique was observed and evaluated using the checklist of six criteria, followed by an asthma education session that included MDI administration technique. The nurse asked the children to demonstrate exactly how they use their inhalers at home using their own MDI devices. The inhalers were fitted with a placebo-medication canister to prevent the child from inhaling actual medication during the observation and teaching sessions. Use of the children's own MDI dispenser ensured that their usual technique was being evaluated.

After assessing the child's MDI technique, the nurse reviewed and demonstrated accurate MDI technique. The nurse then guided the child through the correct steps. Depending on the type of MDI being used, if a child was not currently using a spacer one was provided.

At a second session 1 to 4 weeks later, the children's MDI technique was once again observed and evaluated using the same checklist. After the posttest, the asthma-education session and MDI administration techniques were reviewed.

Data analysis

Demographic data, asthma characteristics, and the pre- and post-intervention data were first analyzed descriptively using means and standard deviations or frequency distributions, as appropriate for the level of measurement. The total number of correct behaviors from among the six criteria was determined for both pre- and posttest observations. Differences between pre- and posttest measures for each of the six individual behaviors were assessed using the McNemar test, which determines differences in paired, dichotomous data. The Wilcoxon signed-rank test, which determines changes in paired, ordinal data, was used to determine if there was a difference in the total number of correct behaviors between pre- and posttest. These nonparametric tests for paired data were necessary because the data were not normally distributed and each child's response was linked (pre- versus posttest response). Change in the subjective assessment of the MDI technique's overall quality was also determined using the Wilcoxon signed-rank test. The data were analyzed using SAS for Windows, version 8.2 (SAS Institute, Inc., Cary, North Carolina) and an α level of 0.05 was used throughout.

Results

Ninety-two percent of the children evaluated used their MDI incorrectly (ie, fair to poor) during the pretest; however, less than one fifth of the participants (19%, n = 7) exhibited incorrect MDI technique after the intervention (Fig. 1). The most common mistakes in the pretest included: (1) not holding breath for at least 10 seconds after actuation (56%), (2) not waiting at least 1 minute between inhalations (50%), (3) inadequately shaking the medication (42%), (4) not inhaling fully (42%), and (5) not using a spacer (22%) (Fig. 2). The pre- and postassessment scores reveal a significant improvement in MDI technique, according to the Wilcoxon signed-rank test results ($P < .0001$).

The shake, inhale, and held breath technique-error data that were evaluated by the McNemar tests were all highly significant, with $P < 0.005$

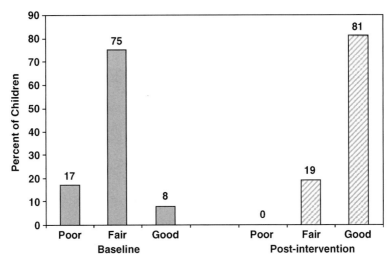

Fig. 1. Pre- and postintervention assessment of children's MDI administration technique (N = 36).

for each comparison. In each instance, fewer participants went from correct at baseline to incorrect at postassessment, compared with those who went from incorrect to correct. Therefore, it is clear that training caused a significant shift from incorrect technique to correct technique for these three criteria. It was not possible to statistically compare the criteria of waiting between inhalations, use of a spacer, and pre- and postintervention coordination, because every child in the study correctly performed these steps during the postintervention evaluation. The McNemar comparison

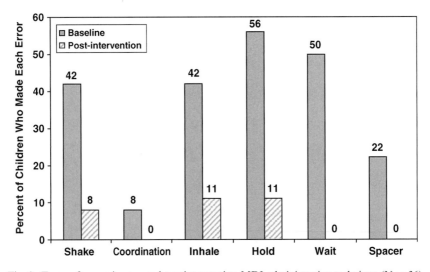

Fig. 2. Types of errors in pre- and postintervention MDI administration technique (N = 36).

requires that at least one participant is in each category (ie, correct or incorrect) at both pre- and postintervention assessment. However, a clear shift in did occur in technique, because half of the children did not wait between inhalations, approximately one fourth did not use a spacer, and 8% lacked coordination in MDI administration during the baseline evaluation.

Discussion

The results of this study were consistent with prior studies of MDI technique in children. The majority of the children used incorrect technique, although they had been diagnosed with persistent asthma and needed to use an MDI for an average of 5 years. Educating pediatric patients and their parents about the proper use of an inhaler significantly increased the frequency of good technique (8% of children before teaching versus 81% after teaching). However, approximately one fifth of the children still used their MDI incorrectly even after training and even though only a short time elapsed between the pre- and postintervention assessments. Despite education and training, 50% of patients with poor technique return to their old habits or develop new errors over time [6].

Parents may not even be aware that their child's MDI technique is incorrect, or may not be adequately supervising them. Winkelstein and colleagues [13] assessed the inhalation technique for a group of school-age children (N = 30) and found that only 7% had effective MDI technique, even though 60% of the parents rated their child's technique as excellent. Ninety-three percent of the children (n = 28) were using their inhalers at home without adult supervision.

The sample's characteristics are a limitation of the present study. The sample was 97% Caucasian, primarily from two-parent, middle- to high-income families, and most were considered to have good to very good asthma control. Six of the 42 subjects did not remember to bring their medication dispensers, and therefore could not participate. Children who have less supervision and who cannot remember to bring their medication may respond differently to the intervention.

Implications for practice

The results of this study underscore the critical importance of clinicians reinforcing medication delivery technique with children and their families at every visit. Parents and children need to understand how, when, and why they take their medicines and should have the opportunity to practice and review their technique with the health care provider.

New medication administration devices

New asthma administration delivery devices are being developed to be compliant with the 1996 US Government ban on chlorofluorocarbon (CFC) propellants. Although MDIs with CFC (Fig. 3) are safe for patients to inhale, they are harmful to the environment because they deplete the ozone layer which surrounds and protects the earth from harmful rays [14]. Therefore, CFC, which is used not only in MDIs but also in air conditioners, refrigerators, and so forth, is being replaced by environmentally safe CFC-free propellants. Medications were given a temporary exemption through year 2005 until a viable alternative for CFC could be found [14]. These alternatives include MDIs containing a new type of propellant, and dry powder inhalers. With the release of new asthma medication administration devices, practitioners are required to learn new techniques and effectively teach them to their patients.

Metered-dose inhalers

Hydrofluoroalkane (HFA) is a new propellant, used as an alternative to CFC in some MDIs. HFA has been effective in delivering beta-agonists, cromolyn, and inhaled corticosteroids [15]. The steps involved in using an MDI with HFA (Fig. 4) are identical to those used for an MDI with CFC. The National Heart, Lung, and Blood Institute [3] recommends the following steps:

1. The canister should be "primed" by spraying the MDI in the air one or two times before first use.
2. Stand up or sit upright.
3. Insert the MDI mouthpiece into the spacer.
4. Shake the MDI and spacer unit vigorously.
5. Exhale.

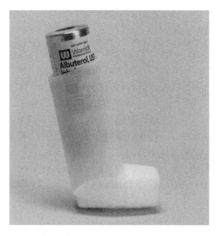

Fig. 3. Metered dose inhaler with CFC. (Courtesy of Michael J. Schumacher, MB, FRACP, UPI Allergy/Immunology Clinic, Tucson, AZ.)

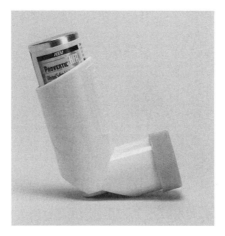

Fig. 4. Metered dose inhaler with HFA. (Courtesy of Michael J. Schumacher, MB, FRACP, UPI Allergy/Immunology Clinic, Tucson, AZ.)

6. Place your lips around the spacer mouthpiece and form a seal, keeping your teeth and tongue out of the way.
7. Press down on the MDI canister.
8. Inhale slowly and deeply through mouth for 3 to 5 seconds without triggering the spacer's warning signal (indicating that the inhalation is inadequate or too fast).
9. Hold your breath for 10 seconds.
10. Remove the MDI with spacer from mouth and exhale slowly.
11. Wait at least 20 to 30 seconds between inhalations.
12. Rinse your mouth after each use.

Breath-actuated MDIs (Fig. 5) eliminate the need for coordination of actuation and inhalation and do not require the use of a spacer. According to 3M [16], the steps for using this type of MDI include:

1. Stand up or sit upright.
2. Remove the cover on the mouthpiece.
3. Locate the up arrow.
4. Hold the canister upright (with arrow pointing upward).
5. Raise the lever until you hear a snap.
6. Shake the canister while continuing to hold it in an upright position.
7. Exhale fully.
8. Place the mouthpiece between your lips and form a good seal, keeping your tongue and teeth out of the way.
9. Inhale with a steady and moderate force.
10. Hear a click and feel a puff.
11. Continue to inhale fully.
12. Hold your breath for 10 seconds.
13. Remove the MDI from your mouth and exhale slowly.

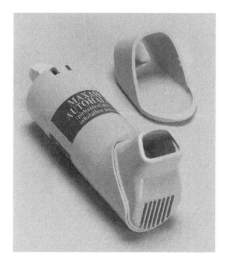

Fig. 5. Breath-actuated inhaler. (Courtesy of Michael J. Schumacher, MB, FRACP, UPI Allergy/Immunology Clinic, Tucson, AZ.)

14. Continue to hold the canister upright and lower the lever.
15. Rinse your mouth after each use.

Dry powder inhalers

Another asthma medication administration device is the dry powder inhaler (DPI). A propellant is not necessary to deliver medication from a DPI because when the patient inhales deeply, the medication becomes aerosolized. However, patients with low inspiratory flow may not get the same amount of drug delivered to their airways as patients with a higher inspiratory flow rate [15]. Therefore, patients who were previously taught to inhale slowly with the MDI will need to be taught to inhale more forcefully to aerosolize the dry powder medication. Also, patients often do not sense the dry powder medication when it is inhaled and may make the mistake of double dosing. A major differences between the MDI and the DPI is that there is no need to shake the DPI.

A Turbutester device, which whistles if the patient inspires with enough force to actuate a DPI, can be used by the clinician to determine if a patient has a sufficient inspiratory flow rate to deliver the medication effectively. However, many patients with asthma who were accustomed to using a spacer with their MDI identify a whistle with inhaling too fast. Depending on the type of inhaler prescribed (eg, MDI or DPI), patients may require additional teaching to ensure they understand when a whistle should or should not occur.

Patients also need to be taught that extreme temperatures and humidity can affect a DPI's drug delivery [15]. All dry powder inhalers need to be kept away from water and moisture to prevent the medication from congealing. Therefore, DPIs should not be kept in the bathroom or in a car's glove compartment, and the patient must be instructed not to exhale into the DPI because the moisture could congeal the powder [15].

Each DPI medication delivery device requires specific techniques for maximal drug delivery. For example, the Turbuhaler (AstraZeneva, Wilmington, Delaware) (Fig. 6) requires the following steps to ensure accurate technique [17]:

1. Stand up or sit upright.
2. Hold the Turbuhaler in the upright position (mouthpiece up).
3. Twist and lift off the cover.
4. Twist the bottom grip to the right as far as it will go.
5. Twist the bottom grip to the left until you hear it click.
6. [Before first use, the device needs to be "primed" by twisting right to left a second time].
7. Face away from the Turbuhaler and breathe out as much air as possible.
8. Place the Turbuhaler mouthpiece between your lips and form a good seal, keeping tongue and teeth out of the way.
9. Hold the device in a horizontal position.
10. Inhale forcefully and deeply.
11. Hold your breath for 10 seconds.
12. Replace the cover.
13. Rinse your mouth after each use.

Various add-ons are available for some of the new devices, such as a dose counter that cues patients when the medication canister is empty. This option eliminates the need for patients to track doses and determine whether medication is present in the canister by shaking or floating it in water. The

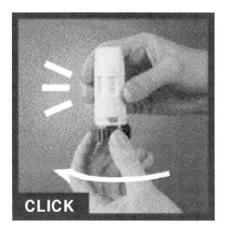

Fig. 6. Turbuhaler. (Courtesty of AstraZeneca LP, Wilimington, DE.)

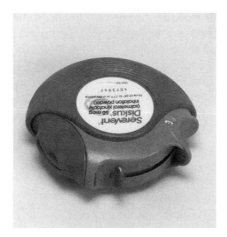

Fig. 7. Diskus inhaler. (Courtesy of Michael J. Schumacher, MB, FRACP, Tucson, AZ.)

Turbuhaler has a window with a red mark to indicate when 20 doses are remaining and when the inhaler is empty [17].

Diskus inhalers (Fig. 7) provide the benefit of a built-in dose counter that indicates the number of doses remaining. The following steps should be performed by the patient using a diskus inhaler[18]:

1. Stand up or sit upright.
2. Snap the mouthpiece into place by holding the diskus in one hand, placing the thumb of the other hand on the grip and pushing away until the mouthpiece appears and snaps into position.
3. Hold the diskus in a level position.
4. Slide the lever away from you as far as it will go until it clicks.
5. Turn your head away and exhale.
6. Put the mouthpiece to your lips and make a seal, keeping your teeth and tongue out of the way.
7. Inhale deeply through the diskus.
8. Hold your breath for about 10 seconds.
9. Close the diskus.
10. Rinse your mouth after each use.

Selection of the appropriate medication delivery system

How is a practitioner to determine what type of asthma medication delivery device to choose? A critical consideration is the child's age. Child and colleagues [19] found that more than one third of school-age children (N = 1444) had been prescribed an inhaler that was inappropriate for their age. Infants and young children 4 years and younger need a facemask along with a spacer when using an MDI [3,4]. For children over 4 years of age and adults, spacers or holding chambers are recommended for all MDIs (except the breath-actuated device) to ensure distribution of the medication to the lower airways [4]. Studies indicate that children's length of stay in the emergency department is significantly shorter when a spacer or holding chamber is used with β_2-agonists [20].

For adults and children older than 5 years, practitioners may prescribe a breath-actuated MDI or a DPI [4,8]. The British Thoracic Society recommends only using a breath-actuated MDI for patients who can inhale deeply enough to activate the medication [21]. Therefore, the breath-actuated device may be inadequate during an acute asthma episode [19] when it is difficult for patients to take a deep inhalation or for children with low inspiratory volumes [8]. DPIs require less coordination between actuation and inhalation and do not need a spacer, and are therefore an alternative choice for children over 5 years of age who have difficulty with the coordination of an MDI or are unwilling to use an MDI with a spacer [4]. Clinicians should be aware that giving different types of delivery devices (eg, a DPI for an inhaled corticosteroid and an MDI for a rescue β_2-agonist) could confuse patients and lead to incorrect use. This is because the MDI requires a slow, deep inspiration, whereas the DPI requires a more rapid, forceful inhalation [15].

Commitment to treatment also needs to be considered, given that medication adherence is about 50% [22]. Children's adherence to inhaled medications is lower than for oral medications (eg, 73% for theophylline tablets versus 30% for inhaled corticosteroids) [23]. This may be attributable to the ease of administration of the oral medication and fear of side effects for certain inhaled medications, such as corticosteroids. Therefore, practitioners must consider the likelihood of the child actually taking the medication. A less efficacious medication that is taken most of the time may be more effective at controlling symptoms and inflammation than a more efficacious medication that is taken only some of the time.

Patient preference also is a consideration. Some patients prefer the MDI to the DPI [24] and therefore may be more adherent when the desired method is prescribed. Future research should focus on determining what factors prompt adherence and what interventions can be taken to ensure consistent medication usage. There is conflicting data about whether decreasing the number of daily inhalations increases adherence [25]. Practitioners must continue to stress the importance of continuing to take asthma-symptom–controller medications even in the absence of symptoms.

Summary

Regardless of the medication delivery system, health care providers need to teach accurate medication administration techniques to their patients, educate them about the particular nuances of the prescribed delivery system (eg, proper storage), and reinforce these issues at each health encounter. A single instruction session is not sufficient to maintain appropriate inhaler techniques for patients who require continued use [26]. Providing written steps for the administration technique is helpful so that the patient can refer to them later when using the medication.

The National Heart, Lung, and Blood Institute's [27] "Practical Guide for the Diagnosis and Management of Asthma" recommends that practitioners follow these steps for effective inhaler technique training when first prescribing an inhaler:

1. Teach patients the steps and give written instruction handouts.
2. Demonstrate how to use the inhaler step-by-step.
3. Ask patients to demonstrate how to use the inhaler. Let the patient refer to the handout on the first training. Then use the handout as a checklist to assess the patient's future technique.
4. Provide feedback to patients about what they did right and what they need to improve. Have patients demonstrate their technique again, if necessary.

The last two steps should be performed (ie, demonstration and providing feedback on what patients did right and what they need to improve) at every subsequent visit. If the patient makes multiple errors, it is advisable to focus on improving one or two key steps at a time.

With improvements in drug delivery come challenges, necessitating that practitioners stay current with new medication administration techniques. Teaching and reinforcing accurate technique at each health care encounter are critical to help ensure medication efficacy for patients with asthma. Since one fifth of children in the study performed incorrect medication technique even after education, checklists of steps for the correct use of inhalation devices, such as those provided in this article, should be given to patients for home use and for use by clinicians to evaluate patient technique at each health encounter.

Acknowledgments

This work was supported by Grant # NUR-017 from GlaxoSmithKline (Clinical Applications Research) awarded to Dr. Burkhart. The authors gratefully acknowledge the critical review of the manuscript by Dr. Lynne Hall, Assistant Dean for Research and the PhD Program, College of Nursing, University of Kentucky. The research was presented as a paper presentation at the Southern Nursing Research Society Conference in Louisville, KY in February 2004.

References

[1] Centers for Disease Control and Prevention. National Center for Health Statistics: asthma prevalence, health care use and mortality, 2000–2001. Available at: http://www.cdc.gov/nchs/products/pubs/pubd/hestats/asthma/asthma.htm. Accessed Januaty 2, 2004.

[2] American Lung Association. Trends in asthma morbidity & mortality. Available at: http://www.lungusa.org/data/asthma/ASTHMAdt.pdf. Accessed January 2, 2004.

[3] National Heart, Lung, and Blood Institute. Guidelines for the diagnosis and management of asthma: expert panel report 2. Bethesda, MD: National Institutes of Health; 1997. Washington, DC, US Department of Health and Human Services, Publication #97-4051.

[4] O'Callaghan C, Barry PW. How to choose delivery devices for asthma. Arch Dis Child 2000; 82(3):185-7.

[5] Scarfone RJ, Capraro GA, Zorc JJ, et al. Demonstrated use of metered-dose inhalers and peak flow meters by children and adolescents with acute asthma exacerbations. Arch Pediatr Adolesc Med 2002;156(4):378-83.

[6] McFadden ER Jr. Improper patient techniques with metered dose inhalers: clinical consequences and solutions to misuse. J Allergy Clin Immunol 1995;96(2):278-83.

[7] Ingram RH. What's new in medicine: getting ahead and staying ahead of asthma. Available at: http://www.medscape.com/viewarticle/449541_print. Accessed March 11, 2003.

[8] American Academy of Allergy and Immunology. Pediatric asthma: promoting best practices. Available at: http://www.aaaai.org/members/resources/initiatives/pediatricasthmaguidelines/default.stm. Accessed January 2, 2004.

[9] Buxton LJ, Baldwin JH, Berry JA, et al. The efficacy of metered-dose inhalers with a spacer device in the pediatric setting. J Am Acad Nurse Pract 2002;14(9):390-7.

[10] Burkhart PV, Dunbar-Jacob JM, Rohay JM. Accuracy of children's self-reported adherence to treatment. J Nurs Scholarsh 2001;33(1):27-32.

[11] Burkhart PV, Dunbar-Jacob JM, Fireman P, et al. Children's adherence to recommended asthma self-management. Pediatr Nurs 2002;28(4):409-14.

[12] Hughes DM, McLeod M, Garner B, et al. Controlled trial of a home and ambulatory program for asthmatic children. Pediatrics 1991;87(1):54-61.

[13] Winkelstein ML, Huss K, Butz A, et al. Factors associated with medication self-administration in children with asthma. Clin Pediatr (Phila) 2000;39(6):337-45.

[14] National Heart, Lung, and Blood Institute. Your metered-dose inhaler will be changing...here are the facts. Available at: http://www.nhlbi.nih.gov/health/public/lung/asthma/mdiintro.htm. Accessed January 2, 2004.

[15] Casale TB. Waiting to inhale: new approaches to drug delivery. Presented at the 96th International Conference of the American Thoracic Society. Toronto (Ontario), May 5-10, 2000.

[16] 3M Pharmaceuticals. Maxair autohaler: patient instructions for use video. Available at: http://www.3m.com/us/healthcare/pharma/maxair/maxair_pt_instr_160x120_avi.jhtml. Accessed January 2, 2004.

[17] AstraZeneca. Pulmicort Turbuhaler [instructions for use]. Wilmington, DE: AstraZeneca Pharmaceuticals; 2000.

[18] GlaxoSmithKline. How to use the Advair Diskus. Triangle Park, NC: GlaxoSmithKline; 2001.

[19] Child F, Davies S, Clayton S, et al. Inhaler devices for asthma: do we follow the guidelines? Arch Dis Child 2002;86(3):176-9.

[20] Cates CC, Bara A, Crilly JA, et al. Holding chambers versus nebulisers for beta-agonist treatment of acute asthma. Cochrane Database Syst Rev 2003;(3):CD000052.

[21] British guidelines on asthma management 1995. Review and position statement. Thorax 1997;52(Suppl 1):S1-21.

[22] Burkhart P, Dunbar-Jacob J. Adherence research in the pediatric and adolescent populations: a decade in review. In: Hayman L, Mahon M, Turner J, editors. Chronic illness in children: an evidence-based approach. New York: Springer; 2002. p. 199-229.

[23] Kelloway JS, Wyatt RA, Adlis SA. Comparison of patients' compliance with prescribed oral and inhaled asthma medications. Arch Intern Med 1994;154(12):1349-52.

[24] Ram FS, Wright J, Brocklebank D, et al. Systematic review of clinical effectiveness of pressurised metered dose inhalers versus other hand held inhaler devices for delivering beta (2)agonists bronchodilators in asthma. BMJ 2001;323(7318):901–5.

[25] Cochrane MG, Bala MV, Downs KE, et al. Inhaled corticosteroids for asthma therapy: patient compliance, devices, and inhalation technique. Chest 2000;117(2):542–50.

[26] Kamps AW, Brand PL, Roorda RJ. Determinants of correct inhalation technique in children attending a hospital-based asthma clinic. Acta Paediatr 2002;91(2):159–63.

[27] National Heart, Lung, and Blood Institute. Practical guide for the diagnosis and management of asthma. Available at: http://www.nhlbi.nih.gov/health/prof/lung/asthma/practgde.htm. Accessed January 2, 2004.

ELSEVIER
SAUNDERS

Nurs Clin N Am 40 (2005) 183–189

NURSING
CLINICS
OF NORTH AMERICA

Index

Note: Page numbers of article titles are in **boldface** type.

Changing Your Address?

Make sure your subscription changes too! When you notify us of your new address, you can help make our job easier by including an exact copy of your Clinics label number with your old address (see illustration below.) This number identifies you to our computer system and will speed the processing of your address change. Please be sure this label number accompanies your old address and your corrected address—you can send an old Clinics label with your number on it or just copy it exactly and send it to the address listed below.

We appreciate your help in our attempt to give you continuous coverage. Thank you.

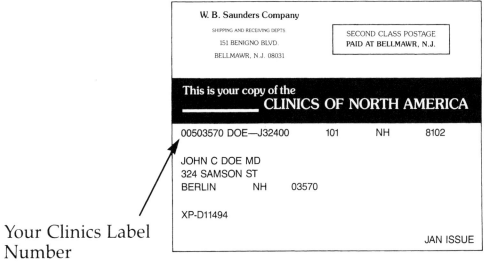

W. B. Saunders Company

SHIPPING AND RECEIVING DEPTS.
151 BENIGNO BLVD.
BELLMAWR, N.J. 08031

SECOND CLASS POSTAGE
PAID AT BELLMAWR, N.J.

This is your copy of the
_____ **CLINICS OF NORTH AMERICA**

00503570 DOE—J32400   101   NH   8102

JOHN C DOE MD
324 SAMSON ST
BERLIN   NH   03570

XP-D11494

JAN ISSUE

Your Clinics Label Number

Copy it exactly or send your label along with your address to:
W.B. Saunders Company, Customer Service
Orlando, FL 32887-4800
Call Toll Free 1-800-654-2452

Please allow four to six weeks for delivery of new subscriptions and for processing address changes.